Head

THE CommonSense

APPROACH

Pat Thomas

Newleaf

Newleaf

an imprint of
Gill & Macmillan Ltd
Goldenbridge
Dublin 8
with associated companies throughout the world
www.gillmacmillan.ie
© Pat Thomas 1999
0 7171 2923 3
Index compiled by Helen Litton
Design by Identikit Design Consultants, Dublin
Print origination by Carole Lynch
Printed by ColourBooks Ltd, Dublin

This book is typeset in Revivial565 9.5pt on 15pt.

A CIP catalogue record for this book is available
from the British Library.

1 3 5 4 2

Contents

While the author has made every effort to ensure that the information contained in this book is accurate, it should not be regarded as an alternative to professional medical advice. Readers should consult their general practitioners or physicians if they are concerned about aspects of their own health, and before embarking on any course of treatment. Neither the author, nor the publishers, can accept responsibility for any health problem resulting from using, or discontinuing, any of the drugs described here, or the self-help methods described.

CHAPTER 1

What are Headaches?

Headaches are among the oldest and most common health complaints of the human race. Their subtle and not-so-subtle levels of pain can range from the dull throbbing of a tension headache to the nausea, flashing lights and drilling sensation of a classic migraine. The pain can last minutes, hours or even days; it can debilitate or even, according to legend, inspire.

For instance, it is theorised that the flashing light in the conversion of Saul to Paul in the Bible story may have been a migraine aura. In later years, Paul became a great manager, preacher and writer, transcending the often painful bouts of headache and visual problems which would plague him for the rest of his life.

The weird trip that Alice took in Wonderland gave her a headache. But could Lewis Carroll, also a migraine sufferer, ever have imagined that one day other migraine sufferers would be described as experiencing an 'Alice in Wonderland' syndrome — feeling parts of their body growing or shrinking to odd shapes and sizes and seeing things which are not there?

Although we tend to think of headaches as a result of modern life, this is not the case. The search for a cure for headaches has a long history. In the Stone Age, it is believed that pieces of a headache sufferer's skull were cut away with flint instruments in order to relieve pain. The ancient Egyptians blamed head pain on invasion by evil spirits and treated it with a mixture of herbs, including opium. Hippocrates, the father of modern medicine, described clearly the course of migraine in 400BC.

Around the time of the birth of Christ, physicians bled their already long-suffering patients and then applied a hot iron to the site of the pain. They also made incisions in the temple into which they inserted raw garlic. When that failed they sometimes tried applying electric eels (living and dead) directly to the head. Two centuries later in Alexandria, the physician Aretaeus added his own description of migraine to the mix, though he labelled it hemicrania in an attempt to describe its one-sided effect.

Around the ninth century in the British Isles, one headache remedy involved drinking the juice of elderseed, cow's brain and goat's dung dissolved in vinegar. It sounds pretty unpleasant, but couldn't have been much worse than the side-effects of some modern remedies. One of the newest class of headache drugs can cause severe chest pain and tightness and even heart attack, flushing, dizziness, weakness, altered liver function, nausea and vomiting. Another common remedy given to migraine sufferers can cause similar effects and has even been shown to make headaches worse in some individuals. Aspirin, taken in large quantities over long periods of time, can cause dreadful side-effects such as intestinal bleeding and kidney damage.

Today's remedies may be chemically more sophisticated, but we are still a long way from providing effective drug relief from the wide variety of commonly experienced headaches.

Who Gets Headaches?

Almost anyone can get a headache — there is evidence to show that nine out of ten adults have suffered a headache at some time in their life. Certain groups, however, are more prone to head pain than others. For instance, women are three times more likely to get headaches than men. It is thought that in some women normal hormonal fluctuations may be linked to chronic headaches, though this is by no means the only explanation for women's headaches. Other groups prone to recurring headaches include children, whose lives are often more stressful than most adults imagine and who have a much stronger mind/body connection. The elderly are also more prone to headaches than the rest of the population. This is not a 'normal' part of ageing; it may be in part because they are also the group most likely to be taking prescription drugs which can produce headaches as an adverse effect.

A Symptom Not a Disease

While we are still a long way from fully understanding the mechanism of headaches, and thus providing appropriate treatment on an individual basis, what we do know is that headaches, including migraines, are not in themselves disorders but symptoms of some other problem. Find the problem and you will find the solution — or the beginning of one — to your headache pain.

One of the most effective ways to find the problem is to become a headache detective. No-one else can do this for you. No-one else lives in your body, or knows your pattern of symptoms and pain. Believe it or not, not even your doctor will be as expert as you about your own headache. You hold the key, and by making yourself aware of the circumstances which trigger your headache, usually through keeping a headache diary (see Chapter 3) you are on the road to relieving your headache pain and the disruptive effect it has on your life.

Many people worry that headache pain needs to be treated immediately, which discourages them from taking the time to hunt for the sometimes subtle clues as to what is causing the pain. One of the big misconceptions about headaches is that the longer you have suffered from them the more likely it is that there is something seriously wrong with you. Actually, the opposite is true. Very severe headaches, those which come on suddenly and are caused by meningitis, stroke or a sub-arachnoid haemorrhage, are the most dangerous. These are thankfully rare. Long-term, chronic headaches may be painful and disruptive, but they are generally not life-threatening.

Don't Shoot the Messenger

Some understanding of pain may be useful at this point. Pain is your body's way of telling you something is wrong. Usually it starts in the nervous system as a result of irritation or inflammation. Here a complex system of nerve fibres conveys the message of pain to the brain and the brain responds immediately, usually by sending out an instruction for self-protective measures. For instance, if you burned your finger, your brain would communicate an urgent message to take your hand away from the fire; if you stepped on a stone, your brain would say it's time to put your shoes on.

Although pain can be troublesome and cause misery, it is essentially a messenger. When we blast the pain with pain-killing drugs we are, in effect, shooting the messenger instead of listening to the message. Doing this prevents us from taking appropriate and long-term protective action. While there is a legitimate place in the treatment of headaches for most kinds of conventional drugs, there is often a high price to pay for taking them routinely; a significant number of headache sufferers find that when they take drugs they only end up trading one set of distressing symptoms for another. If the occasional headache responds to simple pain-relieving drugs such as aspirin and paracetamol, great. But it is important to remember that these, like all drugs, can only suppress symptoms. They do not address the root cause of chronic pain.

Redefining Stress

In simple terms you could say that the majority of headaches are caused by some form of 'stress'. For the purpose of this guide, stress can be defined as any one of a variety of things. It can certainly have an emotional origin — the first thing most of us think of when we hear the word stress. But this is a very limited interpretation, since stress can have a physical foundation as well. For example, your body can be under stress from a variety of conditions such as the early effects of a oncoming viral infection, the metabolic imbalances caused by food allergy or multiple chemical sensitivity, or the postural stress of a spinal misalignment.

Stress causes tension, and perhaps not surprisingly, 'tension' headaches are the most common type of headache, with nineteen out of twenty of us suffering from this type of headache at some point in our lives. This is a significant point, since our relatively new understanding of the profound effects of stress is an explanation for why so many sufferers don't dig further to find out the real cause of a headache. Figures show that more than fifty per cent of headache sufferers never report their symptoms to a doctor or seek any outside help. If it is 'only' a tension headache, we tend to shrug it off as unimportant. After all, we may reason, modern life is tough and we are all under stress. It's probably best not to complain, just take two aspirin and forget about it.

Even if your headache is not triggered by stress, the chronic pain which a headache can bring can create stress in your life and the problem can become self-perpetuating. Too often in our culture we try to ignore stress and numb the pain, whatever its source, rather than becoming familiar with it. And yet, it is familiarity which eventually allows us to begin to track down the real cause of headache pain.

Why Alternative Remedies?

The truth is, you are probably your own best general practitioner when it comes to treating your headache, since only you will know what the pain feels like, when it generally comes on, and what makes it worse or better. Although many headache sufferers feel as if they have no options and no hope of relief, there are a wide range of alternative therapies and self-help options available. Pursuing these provides two important things: genuine relief from headache pain; and also a sense that you have achieved something for yourself. This latter point is important, since so many headache sufferers feel at the mercy of both their bodies and the medications aimed at controlling their symptoms.

In order to solve the riddle of your headache, you first need to educate yourself about all the potential causes and your options for treatment. Then if you feel you need to, you should seek out those practitioners who believe in treating the body as a whole.

Because headaches are so common, and because conventional medicine has such a poor track record in relieving them, there has been plenty of good research into alternative therapies. Unlike those suffering from more serious disorders, individuals complaining of headache are unlikely to be dissuaded by their doctors from trying methods such as herbs, chiropractic, aromatherapy or homeopathy. Since many doctors feel frustrated by their inability to help chronic headache sufferers, they may even be pleased to see their patients taking the initiative and investigating other options!

This book details many proven alternative approaches to headache pain. Some are intended to provide short-term relief; others will require a long-term commitment in order to produce long-term relief from your symptoms. What binds all these options together is that, unlike many conventional approaches to headache, they are at the very least unlikely to make your symptoms worse or produce a host of new symptoms which are equally unpleasant.

Although you have all the clues to your headache pain inside you, making sense of what you already know can be difficult. This is where an alternative practitioner may prove a helpful companion. Most alternative therapists are skilled in the art of history taking — an art which many GPs have lost or don't have time to practise. It is careful history taking which will enable both you and your practitioner to track down the clues to the cause of your headache.

Having gone through your personal history, you and your practitioner can begin to piece together all these seemingly unrelated bits of information, until eventually the picture of what triggers your headache becomes clear.

Headaches can occur for many different reasons and need to be treated according to their cause. Often a headache is a sign of imbalance, and surprisingly headache pain can also be caused by factors unrelated to the head itself. Pain in the head can be what is known as 'referred pain', caused by digestive disorders or pelvic irritation and transferred to corresponding areas in the head, where it is experienced as head pain. A good practitioner will know this and search with you for the real cause of your headache, instead of just handing you a prescription for something to (temporarily) take the pain away.

Alternative medicine treats you as a whole person. This is important, since a headache is more than a pain in the head. It is not a disease, but a symptom of something else. Finding the something else is what you and your alternative practitioner can do as a team.

CHAPTER 2

What Type of Headache?

Depending on what research you read, there can be anything from three to 300 different types of headache. Why so many? Because headaches are a particularly complex health problem. By putting labels to the many variations on the theme of headache pain, researchers have been better able to understand the many types of headache triggers (though this has yet to yield any long-term solutions). Labelling headache types is not an exact science, however; many of the symptoms of one type of headache overlap with the symptoms of other types. And while most people tend to suffer from one type or another, there are also those who can suffer from several different types of headaches caused by different triggers at different times. An example would be a person who has arthritis of the neck, muscular tension and migraine.

Labelling headache types also creates problems for headache sufferers, since it encourages a particularly unhelpful kind of diagnostic pigeon-holing. So today, instead of treating people as individuals and recognising that while broad patterns exist, each individual responds slightly differently to headache triggers (and some don't respond at all) we treat them as labels, or as headache 'types'.

There is even a good argument that all headaches are related, inasmuch as they all stem from either metabolic, structural and/or emotional stress. Nevertheless, the experience of pain is entirely individual and other factors, such as whether you are able to rest, your work or home environment and even the weather can profoundly affect the course of a headache once it has started.

What follows are brief descriptions of the most common types of headaches. However, as you read through try not to get too bogged down in the labels; look instead at the bigger picture to see if any of the symptoms resonate with your own personal situation. Each section contains a summary of common triggers for each type of headache, which may give you new possibilities to explore as you begin to search for the causes and cures for your own individual pain.

Tension Headaches

This is probably the most common type of headache, accounting for four out of five visits to the doctor. Chances are, if your headache isn't an obvious migraine or a cluster headache, your doctor is likely to tell you that you are suffering from a tension headache. Today, it has become something of a meaningless, catch-all diagnosis which tells you little, if anything, about the origin of your pain. What is more, the name tension headache can be misleading, since to many people it suggests an emotional/psychological root to the problem.

Some doctors use the term muscle contraction headache instead, though this is not much more helpful. A better description would be a stress-induced headache; in this case, anything which puts the body and/or mind under stress can be the cause. This can include repressed emotions, an unsuitable diet, constipation, insomnia, hormonal changes and indoor pollution at home or at work.

Some people experience this type of headache on a daily basis. The pain, which starts at the base of the neck and spreads over the top of the head and onto the forehead, generally comes from contractions of the muscles in the scalp. Often it feels like a heavy weight is pressing down on your head, or a tight band is constricting it. Sometimes not all of the scalp muscles are involved so the pain can be localised to just one area — commonly just above the eyes.

Muscle contraction is the result, not the cause, and anything which causes strain on the muscles in the neck or scalp can trigger this type of headache. Tiredness, unhealthy working conditions, poor posture and staying in the same position for long periods of time are all contributing factors. Tension headaches are common after long car or plane journeys and amongst computer programmers, secretaries and anyone who has to work in uncomfortable or poorly designed chairs. As this type of headache becomes more and more common, whole industries of chair manufacturers have sprung up claiming to have scientifically designed, ergonomic seating for home and office. Nevertheless, the problem persists.

Although tension headaches can be caused by a baffling variety of different things, the good news is that once you find the trigger, or triggers, it is relatively easy to stop the pain.

Migraine

A migraine is not a headache, but a whole disease process. Clinically it is defined as a specific disease of the nervous system, which produces a one-sided headache, vomiting and occasionally flashing lights in front of the eye. Roughly one in ten people suffer from this type of disorder, which can disrupt much of your life at home and at work. Women are three times more likely to suffer from migraines than men. Children are also susceptible to migraine, though often they do not suffer them in the same way. In a child, sometimes the migraine is felt in the head and at other times in the stomach (see Chapter 13).

Although migraines can be defined by a broad range of symptoms, they also appear to be very individual, with symptom patterns which vary from person to person. Migraines can be debilitating and come on quickly, bringing with them a range of unpleasant symptoms and a pain which is often described as like having someone drill a hole through your head.

It is a misconception that migraines are an intellectual's disorder — they strike people from every kind of background. Nor are they a neurotic condition. The pain of a migraine comes from the dilation, or widening, of the blood vessels in the lower part of the brain. This is what brings about the characteristic throbbing sensation. Dilation is often — though not always — proceeded by a contraction, or narrowing, of the same blood vessels. It is this which is thought to produce the visual problems which sometimes occur before the actual headache. The alternate widening and narrowing of the blood vessels puts pressure on the nerve endings and causes irritation, which in turn causes the headache.

While it sounds relatively straightforward on paper, these changes occur in response to a variety of complex chemical changes within the body. For instance, it is now believed that migraine sufferers — and to a lesser extent those who suffer from tension and cluster headaches — may have an imbalance in an important brain chemical called serotonin. Serotonin influences our sense of well-being, but an excess of it can also cause the blood vessels to contract. An imbalance of such chemicals within the brain can be triggered by a variety of external factors. Stress is one, but equally, hormonal fluctuations, changes in weather and altitude, bright lights, loud noises, disturbed sleep patterns and pollution all play their part. But more and more we are beginning to see that diet, or more specifically food intolerance and allergy, plays a major part in the development of migraine.

Although we tend to think of migraines as a single entity, there are variations of the type of headache they bring. The most widely experienced form is the one-sided, pulsating headache, lasting between one and three days. This is usually accompanied by vomiting and nausea and a sensitivity to light and noise. Between attacks, the sufferers will usually experience complete freedom from pain and other symptoms. This is the 'common' migraine.

The 'classical' form of migraine displays all the same symptoms as the common migraine, but with what is called an aura beforehand, which can last up to an hour. An aura is an inexplicable feeling or sensation which warns the sufferer that he or she is about to have another attack. Often an aura is accompanied by visual disturbances, which can produce a halo effect around objects.

Some migraines follow predictable phases. There is the *prodrome* phase, where there may be food cravings, yawning, irritability or euphoria; the *aura*, with flashing lights in front of the eyes, blind spots in the field of vision, numbness or difficulty speaking properly; the *headache* phase, during which the pain strikes, along with other symptoms such as nausea, vomiting and sensitivity to light and sound; the *resolution* phase, during which the symptoms begin to ebb and the sufferer is able to sleep it off; and the *recovery* phase, which is characterised by exhaustion and a feeling of being totally washed out.

This is a 'complete' migraine, though not all migraine sufferers experience every part of the cycle. What is more, migraines don't always produce severe pain, are not always disabling and do not have to occur frequently. Some people have weekly attacks and others may only suffer one or two a year. These details are unimportant in diagnosis. It is the symptoms, not their severity or frequency, which define a migraine.

Cluster Headache

A close relative of the migraine, this type of one-sided headache produces a stabbing pain behind one eye with weeping and redness of the eye on the affected side. There may also be facial flushing, drooping of the eyelids, sweating and nasal congestion.

Attacks last between fifteen minutes and three hours and they tend to come in clusters (thus the name) over a period of weeks. Typically, there will be pain-free periods in between attacks, but these rarely last longer than three hours in any cycle. Cluster headaches affect four times as many men as women.

It is believed that cluster headaches are linked in some way with seasonal changes. Most attacks, for instance, occur in spring and autumn, when daylight hours are undergoing transition. But cluster headaches also have a biochemical basis. Anything which throws the normal body chemistry out of balance is a likely contributor. This can include alcohol, heavy smoking, cold wind or hot air blowing across the face, dream-filled sleep and foods containing amines, which can dilate the blood vessels (see Chapter 5).

Sensitivity/Allergy Headache

Sensitivities and allergies vary from individual to individual, and almost anything can cause an allergic reaction in someone, somewhere. Sensitivity headaches usually occur between four and twelve hours after contact with the offending substance. They manifest as a dull, aching, generalised pain. This type of headache is a variation on the theme of tension headache and can be caused by single or multiple allergens.

While a great deal of attention has been paid in the media recently to food-related allergens, less attention has been paid to environmental allergens. These can include passive smoke, car pollution, household cleaning products, perfumes and the gases released from our carpets, wallpaper, soft furnishing and plastic items in the home and office. As our homes and offices become more and more safeguarded against the weather, we seal in these toxins, which can, in turn, cause chronic illness with headache symptoms.

Sensitivity/allergy headaches are among the easiest to cure. Symptoms usually begin to disappear once you have identified the allergen and removed it from your diet or environment. Many people are surprised at how much better they feel generally once this is done. Often they feel an immediate surge of energy and a greater interest in life alongside the disappearance of debilitating physical complaints. In some individuals, however, healing can be slow if there has been a long-term toxic build-up in the body.

Sinus Headache

If you suffer from frequent colds or live in a polluted area, you are likely to experience sinus congestion and the aching frontal pain associated with sinusitis. The sinus headache is closely related to the sensitivity/allergy headache and often they have the same triggers.

The sinuses are hollow, air-filled spaces in the cheek bones and the bones of the forehead. These cavities are connected to the nose via narrow channels, and their main function is to produce mucous for the nasal passages. This fluid protects the lungs by trapping any foreign particles that are breathed in. If the sinuses are irritated, either from pollutants or a cold, they secrete more mucous. This excess mucous should flow down the narrow channels to the nose, but often these channels are blocked and inflamed for the same reason that the sinuses are irritated. Stagnation of the mucous leads to infection and to increased pressure in the sinus cavities. As these are surrounded by bone, they are unable to expand to ease the pressure and become quite tender and painful. This is why sufferers often feel an intense throbbing behind or above the eyes.

The most common triggers for sinus headaches are pollen, dust, cigarette smoke and pollution (indoor and outdoor). But the sinuses can also become inflamed as a result of an allergic reaction, thus you should also consider foods and household chemicals as potential triggers.

Dental Headache

With this type of headache the cause is in the mouth. An abnormal bite, grinding your teeth in the night (often as a result of stress and worry) and dental infection can lead to headaches. The pain is usually felt in the jaw and around the mouth, but can spread to the temples.

If your jaw makes a popping, clicking or cracking sound when eating and/or if pain and tenderness come on after eating or yawning, this is a sign of jaw misalignment. This type of headache is generally less severe than other types. It is treated with corrective dentistry and occasionally manual therapies such as chiropractic and osteopathy.

Eyestrain Headache

The eyes are mostly muscle and they can become fatigued from overuse just like any other muscle of the body. Persistent eyestrain can be caused by working in conditions of poor lighting, or perhaps by the need for corrective lenses. Sometimes they are the result of wearing your glasses when you don't really need to, thus forcing your eyes to remain at a fixed focus for long periods of time.

There usually is only one trigger — overusing your eyes in some way. Eyestrain headache can be brought on by long periods of focused visual work such as working at a computer, doing detailed art work, reading books for too long or in poor light, or working in a room with overhead fluorescent lighting. The one exception to these triggers is that a headache around the eyes can also be a case of referred pain — where the pain travels from one site to another before it is felt — caused by digestive disturbances and misalignment of the spine or joints.

Trauma Headache

It may seem obvious that if you bang your head it will hurt. However, a trauma headache can also be the result of referred pain, and damage to the spine or other areas of the body can end up giving you a headache.

With a trauma headache sometimes there is a delayed reaction, so you may not feel the pain resulting from trauma immediately. But once it strikes it can become a regular feature in your life for years afterwards. In addition, the pain you feel may bear little relation to the injury you received. Even small blows to the head can cause severe, recurrent headaches for a long time afterwards.

Once it does surface, headache pain from trauma can occur daily and be resistant to treatment. It may be accompanied by dizziness or nausea, moodiness, insomnia, fatigue and shortened attention span. Spinal manipulation such as osteopathy or chiropractic are often the most helpful therapies in these cases.

Exertion Headache

As the name suggests, this type of headache usually follows exertion such as coughing, sneezing or a strained bowel movement. One classic example of an exertion headache is the headache which comes on after sex. It may sound like a joke, but the exertion of lovemaking, combined with the muscular contraction of the head and neck muscles during sexual excitement or orgasm, can end up causing a particularly severe head pain.

Exertion headaches are vascular in nature — a swelling of the arteries and veins in turn makes the blood vessels in the head swell. They are fairly easy to treat with dietary changes, relaxation techniques and manual manipulation.

Rebound Headache

Among the elderly, headaches are common — but how often do we stop to consider that these headaches may be a side-effect of medication use, not a symptom of something inherently wrong? When a headache is the result of medication (or the overuse of any substance), it is called a rebound headache.

Medications which commonly cause headaches include those used to treat heart conditions and diabetes.

Overuse of paracetamol can also cause chronic headaches. Ironically, ergotamine, a drug commonly used for migraine, can also cause a rebound effect. Ergotamine is a vasoconstrictor; in other words, it narrows the blood vessels. Excessive use of this drug can create circulatory problems and changes in the heart rate or blood pressure, which can result in more frequent and more severe headaches. What is more, users can become quite dependent on the drug and experience withdrawal symptoms when first coming off it. On withdrawal from any migraine medicine containing egotamine, you may experience quite severe headaches, though these will gradually decrease as the drug clears out of your system.

You can also get rebound headaches as you reduce the toxic load on your body. For instance, it is a common symptom in people who decide to give up caffeine. Foods which contain caffeine constrict blood vessels. The eventual 'rebound' dilation can give you a headache. Rebound headaches are best treated by gradually removing the rebound-causing substance and detoxifying the body. Once your body adjusts, the rebound headache usually goes away.

A final cause of rebound headache is emotional/mental stress. This type of headache is often difficult to diagnose, because it happens after the level of stress has been reduced. This is very common, for instance, in busy executives who seem to cope quite well with their hectic schedules all week and then, once the pressure is off, are incapacitated by headaches at the weekend.

Organic Headache

Although this is potentially the most serious type of headache, it is also the most rare, which is why it comes last in the list. The organic headache is the one everybody fears, but which very few actually have. It comes from brain tumours and in-fections such as meningitis. This type of headache constitutes only one or two per cent of all headaches. This is a serious headache which should be ruled out to your satisfaction before you begin any treatment for headache pain. In general, the pain of an organic headache comes on suddenly, will occur daily and can be made worse through exertion or coughing.

Any new type of head pain which is not relieved by sleeping or wakes you up at night and may be accompanied by bleeding from the nose, mouth or ear should be taken very seriously and investigated by your doctor.

CHAPTER 3

Tracking Down the Cause

All our major body systems are finely balanced and it does not take much to turn bearable stress into unbearable strain. It is the strain of too much stress which inevitably causes our bodies to cease functioning properly and to send out warning signals in the form of headaches and other symptoms.

In order to understand the effect of all these stresses on your body, you must also understand something about your body as a holistic system. This includes some basic understanding of how your body functions and the roles which each of the major body systems — the digestive, endocrine (hormonal) and nervous systems — play in keeping you healthy.

Our major body systems are our most important and effective defences against illness. When one or more of them are working poorly due to outside influences or to poor maintenance by the body's owner — *you* — illness, with headache symptoms, can follow.

The Digestive System

What you eat and how you eat play a big part in your overall health. In a normal healthy person, digestion starts as soon as food enters your mouth. The saliva which you produce while chewing begins to break down your food, making it easier for your body to digest once it reaches the stomach. In the stomach, digestive juices liquefy and process your food further so that it can move into the intestines, where essential nutrients and non-nutrient components are extracted.

Several things can interfere with the process of digestion. Repeatedly eating too much too quickly and eating the wrong types of foods — those which you may be sensitive or allergic to, those which are highly processed and include lots of preservatives and additives, and those which are high in sugar and fat — may cause the system to break down. They may damage the intestinal wall and make it unable to draw nutrients from your food. High and regular consumption of these types of foods can lead to a condition called leaky gut syndrome, where the walls of the intestines which normally act as a barrier and gatekeeper become damaged and begin to let toxins and other irritants into the bloodstream. Once this happens, your immune system becomes over stimulated, acting as if it were under attack by these foreign particles. Many bodily symptoms come with leaky gut, among them chronic headaches.

Even if your gut is more or less intact, poor digestion can mean that you are not absorbing many of the essential nutrients you need to maintain good health.

The Endocrine System

We tend to think of hormones in a very limited way, our perception being that they only govern our sexual characteristics. But the word hormone comes from a Greek word meaning 'to set into action'. Hormones are powerful chemical messengers which guide and regulate most of the body's chemistry, normalising and integrating all our bodily functions. The many different kinds of hormones in the body provide a kind of blueprint, which determines, among other things, how tall we are, the distribution of hair and body fat, how our voices sound, our emotional patterns and the type and location of pain.

When substances identified as toxic enter the bloodstream and begin to irritate the major organs and tissues of the body,

he endocrine system is also affected. It becomes stimulated
nto overdrive in order to assist the process of detoxifying the
ody before it becomes too weak to defend itself.

As a side note, hormonal changes associated with the
menstrual cycle are a contributing factor in some women's
headaches. Many women accept without question the diagnosis
of 'hormonal imbalance' as if it were a normal part of being a
woman. It is not. If you can link your headache with your
monthly cycle, you have taken only the first step. The next step
is to consider all the reasons why your hormonal system may be
out of balance. The cause is likely to lie in diet, environment
and lifestyle rather than raging hormones.

The Nervous System

Although all the major body systems are interrelated, the
nervous system is linked most closely to the endocrine system.
The nervous system is comprised of the brain, spinal chord and
nerve fibres, plus all the chemical messengers which help the
various areas of the body communicate with each other. These
chemical messengers are called neurotransmitters and the two
most important ones with regard to headache pain are serotonin
and endorphins.

Serotonin affects our sense of well-being and also regulates
the diameter of blood vessels, digestive smooth muscle operation, our moods and reactions to stress. Endorphins lessen our
perception of pain and regulate message transmission between
nerves. Other key neurotransmitters which are involved in our
perception of pain include dopamine, norepinephrine and
acetylcholine. When the production and function of these
messengers is interfered with due to some kind of toxic build-
up or stress, headache can result.

Stress Revisited

Broadly speaking, there are three sources of 'stress' — digestive, mental/emotional and environmental — which can stop your body working optimally and eventually cause illness. Ways to deal with each kind of stress are discussed at greater length in the chapters which follow. But an overview may be helpful as you embark on the task of looking for the cause of your headache.

Digestive Stress

Digestive stress is among the most common physical causes of headaches. It can be caused by something as simple as eating a rushed meal which does not get digested properly, or eating something to which you are intolerant or allergic. Overeating may also be an important cause. We live in a snacking society and studies show that many of us consume much more food than we need. Doing this means that we never give our digestive systems a chance to rest and repair. Instead, they are more or less continually busy dealing with the over-abundance of food being processed through them.

According to the Chinese, the head is a compact representation of the digestive system and head pain always points to a corresponding point in the digestive system. In traditional Chinese medicine, the forehead, for instance, is related to the intestines; the side of the head to the liver, gall-bladder and circulation; and the back of the head to the liver and kidneys. Because of the way in which the head is structured, over consumption of 'expansive' foods such as sugar, alcohol and caffeine and fruit juices is believed to result in pain to the forehead or over the eyes. A dull constant pain in the back or side of the head is believed to be the result of 'contractive' foods such as meat, eggs and salt (see Chapter 5).

The typical Western diet is big on quantity and small on quality. We consume far too many processed foods, more protein han we need, and much fewer wholegrains and fresh fruits and vegetables than our bodies require to stay healthy. Fast foods, however convenient, are the fast track to a variety of health problems. The additives used to give these foods a long shelf-life can cause a toxic build-up in your body, and the lack of essential nutrients can cause vitamin and mineral deficiencies. Denied the proper fuel, your body will eventually start to complain.

Some people believe that in order to compensate for rushed meals and poor quality food, all you need to do is take a multi-vitamin and mineral supplement. For some this may literally be their only source of essential nutrients. But if your body systems are not working well and in harmony, it is unlikely that you will be able to absorb and utilise even these prepackaged nutrients to a healthful advantage. Also, many of the nutritional supplements on the market vary in the quality and quantity of their ingredients, making it hard to guarantee that you are genuinely getting all the nutrients you need. The only real solution is to alter your diet to give your body what it needs to thrive and function optimally.

Mental/Emotional Stress

Mental/emotional stress has an equally profound affect on your body. Emotions, even the ones we label as 'negative', are not toxic. But our responses to them can be. Anxiety, depression, repressed anger and a poor self-image can all leave us feeling fearful and vulnerable. When we feel this way, the body responds to bolster us up, often with a tensing of the muscles.

Muscle tension isn't just a meaningless reaction to the 'stuff' that stresses us out. Although it's not widely appreciated, body symptoms often mirror our emotional states. A tensing of the muscles may even serve a genuine purpose in our lives. What that purpose is depends on who you are. For example, tense muscles can make you feel stronger or more powerful; they may act like a suit of armour to protect you from harm;

they may even be the only thing (you think) which is holding you together when you feel like falling apart. The reason why muscle tension is so hard to let go of is because of the purpose it serves in our lives. Often we can't let go until we feel safe again, or until we find a more positive substitute for this painful body armour.

Other physical responses to stress include adrenaline boosts and high blood pressure. All of these things place a degree of strain on the body and the first thing to be affected can be your immune system. Not surprisingly, all of our so-called negative emotional states have been linked in research with depressed immune system function. A depressed immune system can cause the body to react poorly to a number of different situations. Chronic headaches may be a message from the rest of your body telling you that you are very run-down. A depressed immune system can lead to many more serious diseases later on, so if you are getting a signal from your body that you need help, take the hint.

Environmental Stress

Finally, there is the issue of environmental stress, the scope of which scientists and doctors are only just beginning to comprehend. Indoors and out we are subjected to a wide range of chemical irritants and toxins which can adversely affect our health. One of the most common side-effects of chemical sensitivity, for instance, is headache.

Few of us have the choice of living in an unpolluted environment. City dwellers are often obliged to travel, live and work in places where pollution from cars and factories is a fact of life. Nevertheless, many of the substances with which we come into contact on a daily basis are causing a health crisis in our bodies. Even when we cannot see them, pollutants are all around us in the form of car exhausts, pesticides, formaldehydes, radioactive fallout, moulds, dust, cigarette smoke, pollens, perfumes, air fresheners, cleaning fluids and hydrocarbons to name but a few. People who suffer from chronic headache tend to be more sensitive to all these things.

Also, when thinking about environmental pollution don't forget the environment inside your body. Regular use of certain medications can 'pollute' your body and end up causing headaches. The medicines most commonly implicated in headache pain are those used to treat high blood pressure and other heart complaints, diuretics, analgesics, decongestants and other cold medications, oral contraceptives and hormone replacement drugs, antibiotics, antidepressants, appetite suppressants, arthritis medications and those used to treat hearing problems. If you are taking any of these, speak to your doctor about lowering your dosage or switching to a different medication.

The Weather Link

Another influential environmental factor is the weather. Migraine sufferers, in particular, report that their symptoms can worsen according to what's happening in the atmosphere. While some more conservative doctors might think of this as farfetched, there are writings dating as far back as the eighteenth century describing the relationship between weather and migraine. Amazingly, according to the Canadian Medical Meteorology Network, it was not until 1981 that two researchers, Alan Nusall and David Phillips, began a scientific study of the effects of weather on migraine. What they discovered was that wet, windy, cold weather had a worsening effect on migraine, while clear, sunny and dry weather made symptoms more bearable.

A great deal of research has been compiled since then, particularly regarding the role of serotonin in migraine. Nusall speculated in his conclusion that the pathways involved in the weather's impact on migraine are connected with the body's chemical 'pain messengers' such as serotonin, prostaglandins and various other hormonal agents.

In one study of the particularly bitter Chinook wind conditions of Canada, women were found to be more sensitive to weather changes than men. In another, when the headache diaries of thirteen patients were analysed, Chinook winds increased the probability of headache onset, particularly in those aged over fifty. In yet another study, forty-three per cent of those polled cited weather changes as the trigger for their migraine (second only to stress at sixty-two per cent). Strangely, this is an aspect of health often overlooked by doctors, except in Germany where some physicians are known to make use of daily bulletins from the national weather service to advise patients on the management of common health problems.

Keeping a Headache Diary

The point of all this information is to begin to build awareness of potential triggers and how they work. Most of the time we don't think about, or genuinely aren't aware of, the kinds of stress we are under. We eat food automatically, we shut out the unpleasant aspects of our environment as well as unpleasant emotional impulses. This is why chronic headache sufferers may have to learn to become headache detectives.

When you begin to search for headache solutions, one of the most helpful things you can do is begin by creating a headache diary. Over the period of a month or so, make careful records of your headaches. Your diary doesn't have to be elaborate, or expensive — a simple, cheap notebook will do — but what it does need to be is *detailed*.

Consider your headache diary a consciousness-raising exercise, since you will need to record not only when the headache struck, but everything that happened before and after. Typically, this would include things like food you ate, feelings you had, smells, lights and sounds you were exposed to, whether you slept the night before and where you are in your menstrual cycle.

Not only will keeping a diary help you, but should you choose to seek the help of a doctor or alternative health practitioner, it will help them to help you more effectively.

Establishing a Pattern

Below is a checklist of things you should include in your headache diary. The first six items will help you establish if there is a regular pattern to your headaches. The remaining items will help you describe your headache pain and are useful for designing a treatment programme which suits your individual needs.

1) The date and day of the week

You should note whether your headaches occur mainly during the week or at the weekend. Does going back to work on Monday precipitate a headache? Do your headaches fall on certain days of the week? If so, what are you doing on those days?

2) The time of day

Did you wake up with a headache? Did you wake up earlier or later than usual? Does your headache correspond to a certain time of day, such as before or after eating? Did it occur in the morning, afternoon or evening?

3) Where are you in your menstrual cycle?

Record whether your headache occurred during, before or after your period.

4) Where were you when your headache came on?

What was your physical environment like? Was it stuffy, smoky or noisy? What was the emotional atmosphere like? Was there arguing? Was it tense or intimidating? Does your headache always come on in the same type of atmosphere? Be attentive also to things like smells. Have you been around any new carpeting, furniture or clothing — all of which are treated with chemicals? Have you been somewhere dusty, mouldy or musty?

5) What foods, beverages or medications had you taken?

List everything that you ate or drank over the twelve-hour period prior to your headache. Better yet, if you have a history of headaches, keep a food diary of everything you eat or drink. You may find this difficult at first. Eating is so automatic to many of us that remembering can be difficult. With practice, it will get easier. If you are taking any medicines, make a note of when and how much you take.

6) What were you doing?

Your activities on the day your headache occurred may reveal useful information. Was the day unusually stressful, worrying or upsetting? Did you engage in any unusually physically stressful activities? Were you doing something which required deep concentration for a long period of time?

Describing Your Headache

In addition to noting down information on the pattern of your headache, you should also attempt to describe the type of pain you are experiencing. The following descriptive notes will help you establish what kind of headache you are having. These will prove useful once you begin considering suitable treatment.

7) Where is the pain?

Is it always in the same place? On one or both sides of the head, in the back, front, top of the head or all over? Are other areas painful or sore, such as the neck, upper back, eyes, ears, sinus, jaws?

8) Were there any warning signs?

For example, did you see lights, coloured dots, a blind spot in your vision, or experience numbness? Have you noticed any problems with your eyes, or been in a situation where your eyes were under strain? Were you using a computer or doing close work all day?

9) How painful is it?

Try to assess how severe the pain was — mild, moderate or severe will do. Or if you prefer, use a scale of 0 to 10, with 0 being no pain and 10 the worst pain that you have ever had. Is the pain constant or throbbing, dull or sharp, generalised, or in a tight band around the head? Do you sense the pain as a pressure or radiating to other parts of the body? Did your head feel heavy? Did it feel as if someone was drilling a hole in it?

10) Any other symptoms?

Do any symptoms such as dizziness or light-headedness accompany your headache? Do you have nausea, vomiting, diarrhoea, nasal stuffiness or watery eyes? Are you sensitive to light? To noise? To touch?

11) Your mood

At the time the headache began, or during the twenty-four to seventy-two hours preceding your headache, did you become upset, angry, anxious, worried, bored or sad? Or were you happy? Remember that some headaches occur after the triggering emotion has passed.

12) How long did it last?

Make a note of how long your headache lasted and whether it was a constant pain throughout that time or built up gradually to a peak and then gradually subsided.

13) What is your general state of health at the moment?

Headaches don't occur in a vacuum. Do you suffer from hypertension? Are you run-down? Place your headache in the context of the total picture of your health.

14) What made it better?

Have you already found a way of getting relief? Does an ice pack on the back of the neck or shoulder help? Does heat? Did you lie down, take a bath or shower? Did you engage in some recreational activity? Did you take any medication that you found effective?

Your diary should also include any additional comments which might be helpful. For instance, is there any other factor in your headache not covered by these points? Have you already noticed a pattern which you need to note down?

Once you've got to grips with the information in your headache diary, you are in a position to start making connections between a potential trigger or triggers and your head pain. You may wish to take your headache diary and your conclusions to your doctor or alternative practitioner so that he or she can suggest appropriate treatment. Or you may wish to begin a regime of self-help treatments. Even if you have never considered the latter option before, with good information about your individual headache at your fingertips, you are now in a position to choose safely and with confidence from a variety of effective alternatives which are widely available.

CHAPTER 4

Relief from Stress

Stress can produce many different types of diseases. No-one is sure why some people react to stress by getting stomach-aches, others by having asthma attacks and still others by getting headaches. Each of our bodies has an individual weak spot. It may be that people who get headaches are simply more prone to disorders of this type.

Although stress gets a bad press in newspapers and magazines, not all stress is bad. Our ability to cope with stress is part of what has made humans so successful as a species. The problem is that we cope so well with stress that we often fail to notice a build-up of stress in our lives and end up taking on more of it than we can handle. That's the point when stress turns into strain and begins to show itself in debilitating physical symptoms.

Most people have heard of the fight-or-flight response. When a human is under stress the body produces greater quantities of the hormone adrenaline. Adrenaline sharpens our wits, it gives us strength and speed. If we were still cave dwellers, we would either fight the threatening animal or marauding neighbouring tribe or run away. But modern society is more complex. Often we are subjected to stressful stimuli which we can neither fight nor run away from, for instance if you disagree with your boss, or if you work in a shop and are dealing with a difficult customer. Sometimes the stimulus is out of your control, such as rising levels of noise pollution. Yet while society is more complex, our bodies are still much the same as they were hundreds of thousands of years ago. As far as body chemistry is concerned stress is stress. It makes no difference whether the cause is a wild animal or an outrageous heating bill — the response will be the same.

This automatic chemical response to stress creates problems because unused adrenaline can build up in your system. This causes muscle tension and high blood pressure — both of which are implicated directly and indirectly in a number of disabling conditions, including headaches. In addition to making muscle tension more likely, excess adrenaline can interfere with regular sleep patterns; unresolved stress can also result in emotional turmoil, which can cause anxiety and depression.

So much of the time we are not even aware of stress. As adults we have learned to shut it out, and we may not even be aware of the way in which our bodies respond to stress, usually by tensing our muscles. Often, we are so used to carrying on regardless that we never stop to notice that our shoulders are hiked up around our ears or that our necks seem to have lost all mobility. Adults in particular adapt very quickly to these tense postures and carry them around like a suit of armour, defending us against the daily onslaught.

It is not possible or even desirable to avoid all stress, but what we can do is learn to respond to it in ways that are more appropriate to our modern lifestyle. A first step is to allow yourself to become more aware of how stress affects you physically and emotionally. With this knowledge, you can begin to take some control over how you manage stress. You can start putting an upper limit on how much stress you can and will take at home and at work before you need to take a break — even if it is only five minutes to breathe, stretch or meditate.

Anything which puts you under pressure can cause stress and eventually headache. It can come from concentrating on something for too long, from being bored or under-challenged. Equally it can be emotional, and in this respect is often linked to transitional phases in our lives such as moving house, marriage, birth or the death of a loved one. Recent studies have shown that the noise from office equipment such as computers can cause stress.

The best way to remove the headache is to remove the stress. However, if the stress is too great or too much a part of our lives — such as moving house, or a forthcoming marriage — then removing the stress can seem like a tall order. However, there are several things we can do to take better care of ourselves and to temporarily relieve headaches caused by stressful conditions.

Just as being under pressure can cause a surge of stress-related hormones, relaxation can cause a surge of sedative hormones. This has been demonstrated through studies into relaxation techniques, where blood levels of these hormones and also of brain-wave activity have been measured before and after relaxation and meditation. There is no doubt that you can produce powerful chemical changes in your body simply by taking a five- or ten-minute break.

Learning to relax your mind is remarkably easy. You don't need to spend large amounts of money, there is no special clothing you need to wear and you don't need to affiliate yourself with any organisation. You don't need to attend a class, you don't even need to travel. You simply need to learn to cut yourself off from stressful stimuli for as long as it takes to calm things down again. What follows are some quick stress-busting techniques which can easily be incorporated into even the busiest schedules.

Don't Forget to Breathe

How many times have you been told to take a deep breath and count to ten? It's common advice when a person is upset or panicky. The emphasis in our culture is always on getting the air in, even though this is not the most effective way of relieving stress and balancing the emotions. Many practices such as yoga emphasise the outbreath — and with good reason. It is the out-breath that takes toxins out of the body and allows all the muscles to release fully and relax. If you are tense, a series of full outbreaths will provide quick, effective and total relaxation.

Surprisingly, many people find it almost impossible to empty their lungs completely when they first try to do so. Panic overtakes them and they gasp for breath and tense their muscles even harder. You may find that it takes practice to learn how to breathe properly again, but it's worth persevering. Making a hissing sound as you breathe out may help you to steady the breath. As you become better at breathing out fully and in a relaxed way, you can combine breathing practice with guided imagery, perhaps imagining that with each outbreath you are blowing the tension and pain far, far away. Tension headaches respond particularly well to this approach.

Put it in Writing

A simple but effective way of putting worries in perspective is to write them down, so invest in a notebook and pen. Just filing anxieties somewhere other than your mind is often enough to reduce anxiety. Some people make simple lists of all the things which are worrying them. Others find that journal writing, making time each day to write about what they have done, how they are feeling or what kinds of dreams they are having, is a very good way to stay balanced.

Journal writing in particular provides you with the powerful medicine of hindsight. Over a period of time, as you write about your worries, and also as you write about how you have solved these problems, you often begin to get a sense of perspective about the things you experience on a day-to-day basis. Some of them may even begin to look a bit insignificant after a while.

When this happens, it is just a short step to not responding to them in a way which makes you feel ill.

Rock the Stress Away

Remember how nice it was to be rocked on your mother's or grandmother's lap? And have you ever noticed that young children, when they are very upset, tend to rock back and forth to comfort themselves? This instinctive behaviour serves a real purpose. Rhythmic rocking helps to counteract the panic messages being sent to the brain; it also provides a gentle massage to all your stressed-out internal organs. Rocking encourages your brain to ignore many of the panic messages it is getting and slowly your levels of stress will begin to drop.

Many office chairs now come with a rocking mechanism and in the home a rocking chair can become a family favourite to help deal with everything from crying infants to stressed-out executives.

Try Meditation

Meditation is a good way to let go of your worries for a short period of time. Once you become practised at it you can meditate anywhere. Often meditation involves deep regular breathing, which in itself is relaxing.

In meditation, the idea is to empty your mind. When you do this, you leave your worries behind and are making space for more positive and relaxing thoughts. Some would argue, perhaps rightly, that emptying your mind can be difficult to do in a busy office or on a crowded train. This will be true at first. However, the more you practise the more you will be able to take a five-minute meditation break wherever you are.

If your mind isn't completely empty as you begin to meditate, don't worry. Some people take on meditation as if it were just another stressful job. They become very critical of themselves if a persistent thought comes into their heads while they are supposed to be meditating, or if they can only hold onto emptiness for so long before they start to worry about some aspect of their lives.

If this happens to you, don't be too hard on yourself. The best way to deal with intrusive thoughts during meditation is to acknowledge rather than fight them. Some people do this in a non-judgmental way by saying 'thinking' to themselves each time a new thought pops up and then letting the thought go. After a while, it will become easier to have a meditation break in which thoughts don't come intruding into your rest time.

Guided Imagery

Our bodies react to thoughts and images, which is why one aspect of meditation, known as guided imagery, may be useful. Guided imagery is a flow of thoughts that you can see, hear, feel, smell or even taste in your imagination. It is legitimate day-dreaming for adults.

We all engage in guided imagery from time to time probably without knowing it. Perhaps the best example of guided imagery at work in our everyday lives is worry. When we worry about something we allow ourselves to imagine a whole series of 'what ifs'. We follow pictures in our minds of the many possibilities, we check out our emotional responses to each situation, we may even be aware of how our bodies respond, with churning stomachs and racing hearts, as we run through the scenarios of our worries. If you have ever done this and made yourself feel worse, then you have the ability to do this and make yourself feel better. Worrying yourself sick and imagining yourself well are two sides of the same coin.

A useful guided image when you have a headache is to imagine you are somewhere warm, that your muscles are like ice cubes melting in the warm sun. As the sun penetrates deeper and deeper, reaching every muscle, the tension just melts away, leaving you relaxed and refreshed.

Another good trick is to personify your headache — to imagine it as a person or creature. All body symptoms have a message. If you are not particularly good at listening to the language of the body, imagine that it can talk to you in your language. During your guided imagery, make a note of who the character is, what it looks like, what it has to say to you and what you have to say to it. A great deal of useful information can be gained from this deceptively simple exercise.

Of course, you don't have to follow any prescribed guided image if you don't want to. Any image that makes you feel better will do. It can be equally effective to meditate upon a happy, restful or relaxing memory or make up a fantasy of where you would like to be now or who you would like to be with.

Massage

While massage conjures up images of lying on a table or floor mat for long periods of time, even short massages can be of benefit in relieving tension. Many practitioners will come to your workplace and provide short, on-site massage. This is not a frivolity, but a sound investment in the health of the nation's employees. In one study from the USA, the effectiveness of a fifteen-minute on-site massage on reducing stress was measured. Researchers found that after receiving such a massage, individuals experienced significantly lowered blood pressure.

Tension at work, whether from deadlines or uncomfortable seating, can contribute to workplace headaches. If you and your colleagues are experiencing more than your fair share of headaches, perhaps it's time to arrange for a masseuse or aromatherapist to pay weekly visits. A short massage break will do you infinitely more good than a coffee or cigarette break.

Take a Walk

If you are under a lot of pressure, it is particularly important to get regular exercise, as this will help you let off steam and counterbalance the effects of stress. Exercise has been shown in many studies to help reduce stress levels. If you are at work and cannot simply pop out to the gym, make sure that you at least have the time to go out, take a walk, and get some fresh air. In the summer, find a secluded spot and eat your lunch outside.

Get a (Spiritual) Life

For some people, headache is a sign of emptiness. Studies have shown that a commitment to your own spirituality can reduce stress. Where those who do not belong to any formalised religion would meditate, those who do would engage in traditional prayer. The effect is the same — it takes the individual out of themselves and allows them to place their faith in something bigger than their day-to-day experiences. Many of the studies into faith and spirituality and their effect on health show that people who engage in spiritual practices live healthier and longer lives. People who are involved in organised religions may be encouraged by their faith to take better all-round care of themselves. They may be more involved in their families and communities and let go of the belief that life 'should' always be more perfect than it is. Also, they can release some of their daily burdens to whichever higher being they acknowledge.

CHAPTER 5

The Food Factor

If food is giving you a headache, it's probably because you are intolerant or allergic to it or to the ingredients contained in it. Experts now agree that food sensitivity is an important cause of headaches. Where there continues to be confusion and disagreement is over which specific foods are involved.

Some believe it is likely to be wheat, corn, milk, sugars and oranges. Others speculate that foods containing amines — which can cause the blood vessels to contract — are the main cause. Still others suggest that foods with a high copper content — chocolate, nuts, shellfish and wheatgerm — may trigger migraine in some sufferers. In truth, there is a great deal of overlap between potential triggers. For instance, chocolate contains sugar, caffeine and amines. Citrus fruits can increase copper absorption and the food additive MSG binds to it and transports it around the body. Not surprisingly both citrus and MSG are also linked to migraine headaches.

None of these foods, in themselves, is 'bad'. But certain types of food have been repeatedly implicated in recurrent headaches. The fact is that anyone can be sensitive to almost anything and food intolerance and allergy — like headaches — can be highly individual.

When you eat a food which you are allergic or intolerant to, your body reacts just as if it had been poisoned. Symptoms can include nausea, stomach pains, tiredness and of course headaches. There now seems to be little doubt that food sensitivity is a major contributing factor to migraine headaches (see table, pages 41–2). But a migraine reaction is just the extreme end of a spectrum of reactions which may also include tension-like headaches (since the body will be under stress each time you ingest a food which it cannot tolerate). Many carefully conducted studies have shown that when the offending food, or foods, is removed from an individual's diet, headaches and their accompanying symptoms tend to disappear as well.

Take, for example, one famous study at London's celebrated Great Ormond Street Hospital in 1983. More than ninety per cent of children who had severe, frequent migraine recovered once the foods they were allergic to were taken out of their diets. The results were unequivocal and produced a rate of cure which no medication can match.

Among migraine sufferers there is no clear picture of what exact percentage may benefit from removing potential allergens from the diet; research puts the numbers at anywhere from thirty to ninety per cent. Even more encouraging is that the benefit is consistent for each of the three main types of migraine.

There are several methods which you can use to detect a food allergy. At the most technical end of the scale you can opt for a blood test which will look for specific antigens (chemicals produced by your body as a reaction to the allergic components in specific foods). Many people feel that this is the most accurate way to detect food allergies. But while these types of tests are becoming increasingly more accurate, quality can vary between laboratories. These tests usually have to be done privately and the most accurate ones are also often the most expensive.

FOODS MOST LIKELY TO CAUSE MIGRAINE

In the textbook *The Encyclopaedia of Natural Medicine*, considered by many to be the standard reference for natural remedies, authors Michael Murray and Joseph Pizzorno review three studies into food as a migraine trigger. This table is a summary of their findings. The percentages represent the range of individuals whose headaches were triggered by that food. Bear in mind that each individual can have more than one trigger.

FOOD	%
Cow's milk	57–67%
Wheat	43–57%
Chocolate	26–57%
Egg	22–60%
Orange	13–52%
Cheese	32%
Tomato	14–32%
Rye	30%
Rice	30%
Fish (incl. shellfish)	17–29%
Grapes	12–33%
Onion	24%
Soya	17–24%
Pork	17–22%
Peanuts	12–29%
Alcohol	9–29%
Walnuts	19%
Beef	14–20%
Tea	17%
Coffee	15–19%
Nuts	12–19%
Goats milk	14–15%
Oats	15%

FOODS MOST LIKELY TO CAUSE MIGRAINE	
FOOD *(continued)*	% *(continued)*
Cane sugar	7–19%
Yeast	12–14%
Apple	12%
Peach	12%
Potato	12%
Chicken	7–14%
Banana	4–7%
Strawberry	7%
Melon	7%
Carrot	7%

An equally effective way of gauging whether a particular food disagrees with you is simply to remove it, and a range of other likely culprits, from your diet for a period of one month or two. Then, one at a time reintroduce them, monitoring carefully how your body reacts. It is particularly important to reintroduce foods one at a time, since reactions to foods are not always immediate. It can take twenty minutes, but equally it can take eight hours or more to produce a reaction.

While you are removing foods from your diet, be especially mindful of those foods which you really crave — ironically these are the foods which you may be the most sensitive to. You can take out individual foods from your diet on your own, but if you are considering removing a wide range of foods all at once, you should consider seeking the guidance of a qualified nutritionist; you do not want to run the risk of becoming run-down or undernourished in the process.

Other Triggers

There are a range of other dietary factors which you should also consider when investigating a possible link between what you eat and your headache pain. Some of these are more obvious than others and most are the staples of processed convenience foods. Some, such as specific food ingredients and additives like the orange colour tartrazine, benzoic acid, monosodium glutamate (MSG) and the nitrates used to preserve meats, will be listed on the labels of processed foods.

Others, such as 'flavourings' and 'aromas', are more vague. These can be made up of literally hundreds of synthetic chemicals and manufacturers are not obliged to list them on their packaging. You will never really know which of these chemicals is causing a reaction in you. While governments and regulatory bodies claim that food additives are safe, nutritionists believe otherwise. One of the best ways to eliminate potential allergens of this type from your diet is to eat only fresh foods. Processed foods contain too much chemical junk and even if you are not allergic or intolerant to it, it will certainly put your metabolism under stress.

Alcohol

In researching possible dietary triggers for headaches one study found that nearly fifty per cent of those surveyed reported that alcohol was the trigger. Alcohol is cited most often by migraine sufferers as a trigger. It is probably not the alcohol itself which is giving you a headache, so switching to a low-alcohol brew is unlikely to help. Modern wines and beers contain a range of unpleasant chemicals and preservatives, particularly sulphites, which many people are sensitive to. If you are not sulphite sensitive but wine still gives you a headache, try switching to organic wines, which will not have the pesticide content of regular wines.

Amines

These naturally occurring substances are strongly linked to headache pain of all types. Amines can trigger a chemical process which causes the bloodstream to be flooded with serotonin.

The excess of serotonin causes the blood vessels to contract. Individuals who are prone to migraines have been shown to be particularly sensitive to them, and may even have low levels of a special enzyme which normally breaks down the amines in food.

Foods which are high in amines include any fermented, pickled or marinated food, avocados, bananas, cabbage, aubergine, pineapple, plums, potatoes, canned fish, caffeinated drinks, chicken liver, MSG, chocolate, citrus fruits, nuts, processed meats, raisins, ripened cheese, aged meats, yeast extracts, sourdough bread, onions and lentils.

Red wine contains tyramine and should be avoided by those who suffer from chronic headaches, especially migraine sufferers.

Artificial Sweeteners

Health conscious individuals who choose to use products sweetened with aspartame (sometimes sold under the name NutriSweet, Candarel or Equal) may be putting themselves at risk of chronic headaches. In one study at the University of Florida, the incidence of migraine doubled in participants exposed to aspartame. Airline pilots who consume large amounts of diet sodas in order to stave off dehydration on long-haul flights experience more headaches than those who don't.

Aspartame is an excitotoxin — that is to say, it is one of a number of chemicals which have been shown to damage the nervous system through over-stimulation. There is accumulating evidence that this product, which contains the vasodilator phenylalanine, may be a factor in tension and migraine headaches. In one study, more than eight per cent of migraine sufferers found their symptoms were triggered by aspartame.

Aspartame is found in nearly *all* commercially produced sweetened foods such as sodas, fruit juice drinks, yoghurts, chewing gums, ready-made and quick-to-make deserts, candy, ice-cream cakes, biscuits and even some multi-vitamins. If a product claims to have 'no added sugar' it is generally sweetened with aspartame.

Caffeine

Caffeine dilates the blood vessels. Studies show that men and women who consume more than 240 mg of caffeine (the equivalent of four to five cups of coffee or tea) daily are more likely to suffer from headaches.

Be aware that if you choose to reduce or cut out coffee and tea altogether, you may experience a short period where your headaches get worse. Caffeine withdrawal — just like analgesic withdrawal — can cause rebound headaches. Other symptoms you may experience temporarily include drowsiness and fatigue as well as tremors. These symptoms will pass and in a short while you will begin to feel more energy and less tendency towards headaches.

Note also that decaffeinated coffee or tea is not always a solution — for some it can actually cause an *increase* in headaches. Conventionally decaffeinated coffee and tea uses harsh chemicals which may trigger headaches and are certainly not healthy. If you want to try and make the switch to a decaffeinated brew, make sure it is a product in which the caffeine has been removed by a water filtration method and not a chemical process.

Going cold turkey may be your best hope if you are trying to give up caffeine. Try substituting herbal teas, cereal drinks made from roasted chicory or barley and delicious rooibos tea (sometimes called red bush) for your daily cuppa. Your taste buds will soon adapt. In the meantime, watch out for hidden sources of caffeine such as sodas and chocolate.

Chocolate

Reactions to chocolate are probably due to its high amine content, in particular the chemicals phenylethylamine and tyramine.

Both phenylethylamine and tyramine act on the blood vessels. Research into the link between chocolate and headache has turned up mixed results. Perhaps the best way to test your own reaction is to abstain from chocolate for a week or two and then reintroduce it into your diet. If your symptoms get worse, you can reliably believe that chocolate should be eliminated from your diet.

Cured Meats

If sausages, bacon, hot dogs and deli meats give you a headache it is probably because of the nitrate content. Nitrates and nitrites are preservatives which are used almost exclusively in cured meats. Although there is ample evidence that they can cause illness and may even be carcinogenic, no moves have been made to outlaw them. The characteristic flavour of bacon is impossible to obtain without them and there are even moves afoot to allow these risky preservatives into organic meats. You can only avoid nitrates by avoiding the foods which contain them.

Dairy Products

Foods made from milk are a common headache trigger. This may be because of an allergy or intolerance to one or more of the chemicals present in them. For instance, cheese (particularly aged cheese) contains the amines phenylethylamine and tyramine. So does soured cream. The lactase content of milk may be the culprit in some headaches. Dairy intolerance can strike anybody, but is more common in those of oriental extraction.

Monosodium Glutamate (MSG)

The flavour enhancer monosodium glutamate is widely used in processed foods to make them taste better than they would otherwise. Like aspartame, it is an excitotoxin. A number of headache sufferers report MSG as a trigger. Even more worrying is the accumulating evidence that this chemical wreaks havoc in the body in other ways. In studies when rats were given MSG in doses equivalent to that in baby food, they developed brain lesions and other disturbing symptoms.

MSG is found in nearly all processed food, including potato crisps, packaged soups, ready-made meals, meat tenderisers and canned meats. It goes by many names including natural flavourings, hydrolysed vegetable protein (HVP), kombu extract, hydrolysed plant protein (HPP), calcium caseinate, autolysed yeast and sodium caseinate.

Pesticides

Other potential allergens in food are the pesticides and fungicides used during their growth, during their transport and storage and while on display in supermarkets. Few people realise, for instance, that apples may be stored for six months (or more) before they go on display. All the while they will be sprayed with chemicals to keep them looking fresh. In supermarkets today you can find arsenic on your strawberries, DDT on your spinach, cucumbers and peppers coated with a paraffin wax to make them look nice and shiny and bananas ripened with ethylene gas. The range of potentially harmful chemicals you can ingest is simply vast.

If a number of otherwise unrelated produce items seem to give you a headache, it may not be the food but the pesticide residue which is the problem. Washing won't help remove it all; pesticide residue is remarkably stubborn. The best way to test if you are allergic to pesticides is to switch to organic produce and see if it produces the same effect.

The High Carbohydrate Diet

Doctors and nutritionists are always telling us that a diet high in carbohydrates is more healthy. For headache sufferers this is particularly true. A diet based on complex carbohydrates, such as wholegrains, beans, peas and other 'seed foods', has been shown to increase the amount of the amino acid tryptophan available in the body. Tryptophan is converted in the body into serotonin, which is involved in regulating the diameter of blood vessels and enhancing our feelings of well-being.

A high carbohydrate diet can also reduce migraines caused by hypoglycaemia (low blood sugar). Unrefined carbohydrates and strict avoidance of sugars minimise up and down swings in blood sugar, which may be effective in reducing the duration and severity of migraines. If you get headaches when you haven't eaten for a few hours, or if you are diabetic, you might consider asking your doctor to test for hypoglycaemia.

If you suspect hypoglycaemia, it may be a good idea to get into the habit of eating small regular meals throughout the day. Don't binge on chocolate and other empty snacks. Instead, make sure you have a steady supply of wholefoods such as fruits, vegetables and nuts on hand. Apple juice will release sugar more slowly into your bloodstream than other juices. Think also about how you start your day. Highly processed cereals such as cornflakes may not be the best choice. These are usually boiled then baked, and are probably closer to being a simple sugar (which will sharply elevate your blood sugar and then just as sharply drop it) than the complex carbohydrates found in porridge oats and muesli, which will sustain your blood sugar evenly over a longer period of time.

As with all dietary advice, there are exceptions and, frustratingly, some people do worse on a high carbohydrate diet. If your migraines bring on flushing and itchiness or you have classic migraine symptoms, try in addition to a high carbohydrate regime making your diet low in tryptophan-containing foods such as bananas, milk, cottage cheese, peanuts, dried dates and turkey.

Just to confuse matters, a low carbohydrate diet has also been advocated as a headache treatment. This diet is probably most appropriate when headaches are a symptom of high levels of sugar in the blood. As the sugar is metabolised, it can cause a type of rebound hypoglycaemia. Both the low carbohydrate diet and a low sugar diet have been successful in treating this type of headache.

Helpful Supplements

Supplements can never replace a good diet, but for some, taking extra amounts of vitamin B6, magnesium, lithium and/or essential fatty acids may help relieve migraine symptoms.

Women who are particularly prone to migraine may be low in magnesium (though this can happen in men too). Studies with women suggest that symptoms improve once magnesium deficiency has been identified and corrected. It is best to combine B6 with your magnesium supplement to help its effectiveness.

The whole B-complex will be useful if you are under a lot of stress, but you might want to consider upping your intake of B2 (riboflavin) if you suffer from regular migraines. In a recent study, participants who reported between two and eight migraine attacks per month, took a relatively high dose, 400 mg, each day and started to experience improvement after just two months. It was speculated that B2 helps build up the body's energy reserves — which can be depleted by recurring migraine attacks — making recovery more swift. Although riboflavin appears to be safe in daily doses up to 600 mg, you may not wish to take this much B2 unless under the guidance of a qualified nutritionist. However, you can confidently take a good quality B-complex which contains around 100 mg of each of the B-vitamins.

You should also aim to include more essential fatty acids in your diet. Essential fatty acids are divided into two main groups: the Omega 6 group, which comes from such sources as evening primrose oil, borage oil and blackcurrant seed oil; and the Omega 3 family, which comes from oily fish and flax and pumpkin seeds. We need both for good health, usually taken in a ratio of 2:1, Omega 6 to Omega 3.

Boosting the intake of the Omega 3 family in particular has been shown to be beneficial in headache sufferers. There have been studies to show that patients who have severe migraine, and who do not respond to conventional treatment, often respond to supplements of fish oils. You can up your intake with any number of good quality supplements on the market. However, the best and most flavourful way to do this is to increase your consumption of oily fish such as salmon, herring and mackerel as well as increasing seed foods such as linseed, pumpkin seeds, sunflower and flax seeds, all of which are delicious as a topping on salads and cereals.

If you must take supplements, those which contain fish oils may be particularly useful. However, there has been concern among nutritionists that some fish oils may be contaminated with mercury. If this is also a concern for you, you should take supplements which source their Omega 3 fatty acids from linseed, flax and other seeds which are equally as good. Try taking 1000 mg (or the equivalent of around 50–100 mg Omega 3) of fish or seed-based oil daily for six weeks — you may find that it reduces both the frequency and severity of your migraine symptoms.

Expansion and Contraction

If all the information on food and headaches so far seems a bit daunting, consider the system worked out by Annemarie Colbin, American nutritionist and founder of the Institute of Food and Health in New York. Ms Colbin also believes that headaches are a sign of systemic imbalance and over the years has refined her approach to the causes of food-related headaches. She classifies them either as expansion or contraction headaches, with side categories for 'liver' headaches, caffeine withdrawal headaches and others. Her system is based on the ancient Chinese belief that certain foods are expansive and others are contractive, and that an imbalance of these foods in the diet causes imbalance in the body.

Expansion headaches, according to Colbin's system, are usually the result of too much:

◆ Liquid of any kind, including fruit juice
◆ Alcohol
◆ Ice cream and other cold and highly sugared foods.

These headaches can, she says, be remedied in two to fifteen minutes by eating salty, contractive foods which counterbalance their effect. You might try the following:

Gomasio (sesame salt): You can make this by grinding up one cup of sesame seeds, preferably the Japanese kind known as suribachi which have grooves. Add to the half-crushed mixture two teaspoons of salt, then grind well into the seed mixture.
Umeboshi plums: You can buy these Japanese pickled plums in most health food shops. They taste salty-sour. The best brands have no ingredients other than plums, salt, water and maybe beefsteak (chiso) leaves. Alternatively you can buy paste made from umeboshi which you can take a fingerful of when you have an expansive headache.
Brine-cured olives: Just a few may help to ease your headache pain.

At the other end of the scale, contraction headaches are usually the result of:

◆ Tension
◆ Overwork
◆ Heat
◆ Meats and salty foods (especially taken on an empty stomach)
◆ Lack of food and or fluids
◆ Excess mental concentration or physical activity in addition to the above.

These headaches can take a little longer to alleviate in some cases but the following remedies should work within five minutes to twenty-four hours. They consist of something cool and liquid, sweet or sour such as:

Apple or apricot juice: Make sure it is the best quality you can afford, preferably fresh pressed and if possible organic.
Cold unsweetened applesauce (or other cooked fruit).

In Ms Colbin's system, migraines are known as liver headaches and they usually arise two, four or even eight hours after eating a food which unbalances the system. This is why they can be so difficult to link to the offending food. In her experience, these headaches are usually the result of eating fatty foods on an empty stomach, including fried eggs or cheese for breakfast and salads with oily dressings and avocado.

To remedy this type of headache, use the same remedies for contraction headaches. In addition, try:

Lemon tea *or*
Five phase tea: This remedy can be made at home from the following ingredients. Make one cup of lemon tea and add a tablespoon of maple syrup (you can add more to taste if you prefer). Next, add a pinch of cayenne pepper or five drops of Tabasco sauce (these have a cooling effect) *or* ½ teaspoon of fresh grated ginger (this has a warming effect) — be guided by your inclinations. Stir well and drink hot.

Caffeine withdrawal headaches should be treated as contraction headaches. If even after you have gone through your headache diary you are not sure which type of headache you have, you can find out relatively quickly by having a tiny bite of umeboshi plum, or a fingerful of plum paste. If you remain the same or get better, you have an expansive headache; if you get worse you have contractive or liver headache.

CHAPTER 6

Is Your Home Giving You a Headache?

Your home should be a haven where you can rest and your body can repair itself. Unfortunately, many of our homes only further add to the risk of illness. In fact, indoor pollution is now recognised as even more of a threat to our health than outdoor pollution. The cleansers we use in our kitchens and bathrooms — the very ones which promise to make our homes healthier by, for instance, removing 'harmful bacteria'; the pesticides we use on our lawns; the fumes we inhale while cooking or heating the home; volatile chemicals emitted from aerosol sprays, carpets and plastics; and the electromagnetic field (EMF) emitted from all our household appliances can all cause chronic health problems in sensitive individuals.

Indoor air pollution has become a considerable problem in recent decades. Lance Wallace, an environmental expert working for America's Environmental Protection Agency (EPA), conducted a survey of 600 homes in six cities; he found that concentrations of twenty toxic or carcinogenic (cancer causing) chemicals were up to fifty times higher indoors than outdoors.

Many of the chemicals used in household products are highly volatile, which means they easily evaporate and can be inhaled. Others, sprayed from aerosol cans or hand pumps, release a shower of microscopic, easily inhaled particles known as volatile organic chemicals, or VOCs.

Ironically, you are also highly likely to be exposed to harmful chemicals in the home while doing the things you most associate with washing them away — showering, washing dishes and flushing the toilet. Many industrial solvents and contaminants such as benzene and methylene chloride get dumped into our water supply and can easily pass through the skin into the body during showers, baths and dishwashing. More importantly, these chemicals become gases at room temperature and are then easily inhaled. According to at least two American environmental studies, the amount of industrial VOCs inhaled during a fifteen-minute shower with contaminated water is equivalent to drinking about eight glasses of contaminated water. The longer and hotter the shower, the more chemicals build up in the air. Baths also produce this effect, but to a much smaller extent.

There is much you can do to avoid inhaling chemicals in the home. Avoid using all aerosols, no matter what propellant they use. Every time you use an aerosol you will inhale high concentrations of its chemical contents.

Some headache sufferers are very sensitive to dust, but there is another good reason to keep dust levels as low as you can in your house. Dust particles absorb VOCs and increase their concentration in the air. Limit the time you spend in the shower and make sure the water is warm to cool and finish off with a cool to cold rinse. When you shower, open a window to let waterborne chemicals out and close the bathroom door to prevent them getting to other areas of the house.

Bare Wood Is Better

There is now substantial scientific data to suggest that carpeting may be bad for your health. Although many of us believe that we have made great progress since the days of bare wood floors, carpets are constantly giving off gases which can adversely affect our health. Although we have long known this about new carpets, research from the US suggests that even older carpets may still be off-gassing chemicals which can cause illness.

Writing in the *Journal of Nutritional and Environmental Medicine*, Rosalind Anderson reported how she analysed 125 carpet samples ranging from one week to twelve years old. She put the carpet samples in with mice and found that the breathing rate of the mice was immediately decreased. Other alarming symptoms included swollen face, altered posture, hyperactivity, loss of balance, even convulsions and death. In the course of her studies, Dr Anderson identified over 200 different chemicals being given off by modern carpets which are capable of producing a variety of toxic effects. In humans, common reactions include flu-like symptoms, muscle pain, headache, fatigue, tremors, memory loss and concentration difficulties.

Carpets are also very efficient at trapping outdoor pollutants. This is partly because we track these pollutants in from the garden and other places and there they sit, sometimes for years, in our carpets. But it is also the result of using pesticides indoors. The No-Pest strips which we hang on walls and from light fixtures contain the cancer-causing insecticide dichlorvos (DDVP). In America, an EPA report on non occupational pesticide exposure identified at least five pesticides at levels up to ten times greater indoors than outdoors.

If you are headachy and ill at home, maybe it's time to consider bare wood flooring. To protect yourself and your family from pesticides and other pollutants, take your shoes off before entering the house. Pesticides should be used sparingly if at all and only use enough of the product to get the job done. Read labels and look for chemicals such as chlordane, heptachlor, commonly used in garden insecticides, moth and termite proofing as well as for other purposes, and dichlorvos. Better yet, try using some of the organic pesticides now on the market.

Heavy Metal

Metal toxicity can cause big headaches in some individuals. Unfortunately, sources of metal toxicity are all around us. For instance, if you have a mouth full of fillings it is likely that mercury is slowly leaking into your system. Mercury-sensitive individuals will suffer a range of health problems such as allergies, fatigue, dizziness, headaches, nausea and chronic fatigue.

The quality of the tap water we drink is often pretty poor. Filtration processes don't always remove nitrates and other chemical poisons. Also, our water contains many heavy metals, including aluminium and chlorine — both of which are added to some types of water at treatment plants — and lead. Aluminium has been associated with neurological problems such as Alzheimer's disease, and chloride with damage to the blood vessels and anaemia.

Lead is another major metal pollutant and it is all around us. It is a neurotoxin — which means that it can damage the brain and nervous system. In studies on children, lead has been shown to impede their intellectual growth. The main source of lead poisoning in one study in Edinburgh, commissioned by Britain's Medical Research Council, was water. Lead exposure can also cause high blood pressure — a contributing factor in headaches. While water is a main source of lead, we can also inhale it from car emissions.

To avoid heavy metal poisoning, consider switching to bottled water, or more economically a water filtration system. If you wish to go on using tap water, make sure you run the tap for at least two minutes before using the water for cooking or drinking. If you suspect mercury poisoning from fillings, you can contact the British Society for Mercury Free Dentistry to have yourself tested for mercury sensitivity and take advice on having your mercury fillings removed.

Don't use enamelled cookware — a major source of the toxic metal cadmium. Cadmium poisoning has been linked to a wide range of disorders, including chronic headaches. It is also a well known carcinogen. Other common sources of cadmium are cigarette smoke and excessive tea and coffee drinking.

Electrical Sensitivity

Electrical sensitivity is an environmentally triggered illness with symptoms similar to chemical sensitivity. It is only just beginning to be recognised by some doctors and scientists. Throughout our homes and in our offices, we have a number of electrically powered devices which are intended to make our lives easier. It's hard to imagine that these gadgets might produce side-effects which could cause headaches and other health problems. Nevertheless, exposure to electromagnetic fields (EMFs) from power lines, computers and motors affect the nervous system causing symptoms not unlike chronic fatigue.

In a recent survey published by the specialist magazine *Electrical Sensitivity*, headache was among the most common symptoms experienced by those suffering from electrical sensitivity. Other symptoms included fatigue and weakness, skin rashes, confusion and poor concentration.

Another side-effect of heavy EMF concentration which scientists have found is that airborne particles including water, dust and toxic chemicals concentrate close to electric fields. One study in Norway, for instance, showed that they tend to concentrate under power lines and concluded that airborne products are attracted to sources of power. Researchers are now turning their attention to the question of whether other airborne toxins such as bacteria might also be concentrated around electric fields, adding further to their toxic potential.

To limit the effect of EMFs in your home, try repositioning your furniture. Avoid locating beds or chairs too close to significant domestic sources of EMFs such as electricity meters or TVs. Allow at least six to eight feet from such sources, especially for beds. Bedside radio alarms, whether electric or battery powered, should be at least two feet from your head. Don't plug appliances in near your bed and don't use an electric blanket; if you do, switch it off, or better yet unplug it, before going to bed. Remember that electrical fields can be generated even by appliances which are switched off.

In addition to EMFs, the laser printers, copiers and fax machines now common in homes as well as offices, all release volatile organic chemicals into the air when they operate. Where possible, keep the air clean by opening your window when using these machines, or have an exhaust fan or air purifier which contains a charcoal filter (other types do not remove chemicals) installed nearby.

Plastic Fantastic?

Many common household products emit chemicals without our knowing it. Among these is formaldehyde. Because of the extensive use of building materials and furnishings which release it, formaldehyde exposure is almost inescapable in modern indoor environments. The greatest levels are given off by the glue which holds together fibreboard, particleboard and plywood panelling. The brightly coloured plastics which are now used for everything from storage to cleaning and kitchen implements, from waste paper bins to the casings on our electrical equipment, emit formaldehyde. So do new carpets, no-iron clothes, upholstery, foam insulation, latex paint, space heaters, new paper and some cosmetics such as shampoo, nail polish, skin creams and hair sprays.

Although formaldehyde emission decreases with time, high humidity or moisture can increase its release from glued particle-board and panelling. Chronic exposure to formaldehyde has been shown to produce a number of unpleasant symptoms including headaches, memory loss, drowsiness, nausea, dizziness, short-ness of breath, irritation of the eyes and nose and even cancer.

The Toxic Beauty Trap

If you suffer from regular headaches, you may be a victim of the toxic beauty trap. To avoid this, there are several things you can watch out for and eliminate from your toiletry cabinet. Any product with bright colours (striped toothpastes, coloured mouthwashes, shampoos, deodorants, etc.) should be used with caution, since many of them contain synthetic dyes which have been implicated in a number of health problems. Perfumed products should also be regarded with suspicion.

If you suspect that chemical sensitivity is a trigger in your headaches, then it's time to make the switch to cosmetics which are not coloured or perfumed. Remember, neither the colour of the product nor its scent add to its effectiveness. Don't be fooled by products which say they are natural — natural is a highly abused and overused word in the cosmetic and toiletry industry. Usually it means that synthetic petro-chemicals have been used to approximate the real thing. For instance, if a product label says it contains the natural smell of lemons, this does not mean that they have used lemon essential oils to enhance its scent. It is more likely to be a synthetic version made up of literally hundreds of different chemicals. Unless a product lists the proper Latin name for essential oils, they are not using them as a scent.

A Final Word

It is not possible to protect ourselves from every potential irritant in the environment. This is the world we have built and we have to live in it. Nevertheless, if you do suffer from chronic health problems, it is important to try and reduce the *total load* on your body wherever possible. Taking whatever steps you are able to will certainly improve your overall health. For some individuals, it may signal the end of a headache pain which has been plaguing them for years.

CHAPTER 7

Herbal Remedies

While herbal remedies still conjure up images of witches brew to some people (and maybe especially to their doctors!) there is now a great deal of scientific validation for their use. Herbs have long been an essential part of medicine and many of today's synthetic medicines have been copied (not always successfully) from herbal 'blueprints'. According to the World Health Organization, herbal medicine is the third most widely used type of medicine in the world. It is also one of the oldest forms of medicine.

When palaeontologists discovered bunches of herb fossils at ancient dwelling sites, it confirmed a long-held suspicion that medicinal herbs have been in use almost as long as man has been walking the Earth. The uses of herbs were being passed down from generation to generation as part of an oral tradition, long before we began to use books to record such information. Ancient Eastern civilisations used many animal, plant and mineral remedies. When Hippocrates utilised local plant remedies to support the patient's own healing powers, a new interest in preventative medicine grew and herbal remedies continued to be used throughout Roman times. The Persians and Arabs added new remedies of their own and the knowledge of herbal medicine extended to the Western world.

Even as late as the early nineteenth century, physicians were still receiving stiff competition from traditional healers. In

America, the early settlers got some of their most valuable health education regarding native vegetation from the American Indians. By the late 1800s, however, the scientific community began to isolate the active ingredients in many natural substances with the hope that they could eventually be synthesised in the laboratory. It wasn't long before they were.

Herbal remedies can be used alone or to complement conventional care. There are herbs to treat specific conditions, to ease pain and inflammation, relax or stimulate organs, fight bacteria and boost the immune system.

Herbs can be used in many different forms: capsules and tablets made from the dried or powdered plant; extracts where the juice has been squeezed from the fresh plant; tinctures where the plant has been steeped in alcohol, vinegar or glycerine; or teas which can be made from both the dried and fresh leaves, flowers, roots and barks of the plant. Generally speaking, the less processing that has gone into the preparation the more you will benefit from it. This is why some herbalists recommend extracts and tinctures as the most effective way to take herbs. Herbal remedies can be taken internally and applied externally as ointments, creams and essential oils.

Herbs are powerful medicine and should be taken with the same caution and respect you would take with any medication. Whether you are self-prescribing or going to a qualified herbalist, you should be prepared to ask and be satisfied with the answers to certain questions: What is the herb? Is it from an organic source? What effect can I expect it to have? Are there any side-effects I should watch out for? Does it have any adverse interactions with conventional medications?

Herbs for Headaches

Herbal remedies have a number of actions which can be useful in headaches. Tonic herbs can boost the body's own ability to fight off infection — useful if your headache has a viral origin.

They can be used to detoxify the body and so can help in cases of toxic build-up. Herbs can be used to help re-balance hormones safely and some act directly to relieve pain. Whatever type of herb you use, it is important to understand that herbs act more slowly than conventional medicine. The aim is to build health from the inside out and this can take time, particularly if your health has been poor for some years.

Several herbs have shown promise in research trials on headache. Most of these can be bought in over-the-counter preparations from your local health food shop.

Capsaicin

Capsaicin — the active ingredient found in cayenne pepper — is one of the most widely used herbs for headache relief. It can be taken internally in small amounts, but more often is applied as a cream to the site of pain. It is thought that when a cream containing capsaicin is applied to the skin, it works in two ways: by blocking pain signals, and by diminishing the chemical transmitters which cause pain impulses.

The best products are those which contain 0.025 to 0.075 per cent standardised capsaicin. These are generally available in health food shops.

Cayenne seems to cause minimal side-effects. In rare cases, people have reported allergic reactions including rashes. Taken internally, it can cause digestive tract inflammation in some. It appears that these side-effects are most common at the beginning of treatment and that the body quickly builds up a tolerance to the herb. If you are taking cayenne in oral doses, the best way to avoid tummy upsets is to take it with food. Pregnant women should not use cayenne, as it can cause uterine contractions.

Feverfew

Feverfew is one of our most valuable herbs in the treatment of migraine. In all, more than fifty scientific papers have been published in the past fifteen years which examine the efficacy of this powerful herb. One of the most important studies was carried out at University Hospital Nottingham in 1988. In it, seventy-two migraine sufferers were randomly given either one capsule containing dried feverfew leaves or a matching placebo for four months.

Next, the treatments were switched, with the placebo group receiving feverfew and vice versa, for a further four months. The number of migraine attacks fell by twenty-four per cent and significantly fewer working days were lost to headache in the feverfew group compared to the placebo group. The feverfew group also experienced a reduction in the number and severity of migraine attacks and the degree of vomiting.

In another study, when migraine sufferers who regularly took the herb were unknowingly given a placebo instead, their migraines worsened.

Feverfew is best taken in tablet form since the dried leaves can be bitter and with tea there is no way of guaranteeing a consistent strength. The active ingredient in the herb is thought to be parthenolide (although a recent analysis of studies into feverfew at the University of Exeter suggests that there may be other beneficial, but as yet unidentified, ingredients in the whole plant). However, consumers beware. When researchers in Nottingham tested several dried preparations, they found parthenolide levels varied widely between products and was not detected at all in some. Make sure you check the label of any preparation you are intending to buy. It should contain at least 0.2 per cent of parthenolide in every 125 mg of feverfew leaf powder to be effective.

Feverfew is generally free from side-effects. However, certain restrictions in its use do apply. Children under two should not be given feverfew and pregnant women should also avoid it, since it can cause miscarriage.

White Willow Bark

This is probably the original non-steroidal anti-inflammatory drug (NSAID) and has been used as a pain reliever since 500BC. By the eighteenth century, European healers were also employing it to treat fevers. The active ingredient of white willow bark (*Salix alba*) is salicin, which was isolated in 1828. When digested, this chemical is believed to be converted into salicylic acid — the same compound as is used in aspirin.

What makes this herb more appealing than aspirin, however, is that it has been shown to cause less gastrointestinal irritation. Headache sufferers who can't take aspirin because it upsets their stomachs may find that white willow bark, with its lower concentration of salicytes, is more acceptable. The downside is that it will not work as quickly as aspirin. But some other species of willow including *Salix daphnoids*, *Salix fragilis* and *Salix purpurea*, contain higher concentrations of salicin. Look for these Latin names on any herbal pain reliever you buy.

While generally free from side-effects some people experience gastrointestinal upsets if they take too much of this herb too regularly. Pregnant and nursing women should not use white willow bark, since salicin has been associated with an increased risk of birth defects. It should not be given to children under two or to young children with colds, flu or chicken pox, since — like aspirin — it has the potential to cause a sometimes fatal disease called Reyes' syndrome.

Ginger

Ginger is an uncommon remedy for headaches in the West, but in East Africa it is commonly used to treat a wide range of different headaches. Although ginger probably does not act directly on your headache, it can be particularly helpful in cases of migraine where other symptoms such as nausea and vomiting are present. If your headache is accompanied by stress and fatigue, ginger may have the effect of perking you up (without the side-effects of other stimulants such as caffeine) and thus relieve or diminish headache pain.

Fresh ginger root is widely available in supermarkets and you can easily make a warming, reviving tea by grating a teaspoon or two of the root and pouring boiling water over it. Using it liberally in your cooking will also be beneficial. It works equally well in sweet and savoury dishes.

Garlic

This is another widely available remedy, which you might not immediately think of in relation to headaches, and yet garlic has many actions which may be beneficial for headache sufferers. First and foremost garlic helps strengthen the immune system, but it has other beneficial effects as well. For instance, it reduces the 'stickiness' of the blood, helping it to flow more freely. This is why it is often recommended for those with high blood pressure. Garlic has no known side-effects, apart from garlic breath. If this worries you, you can always take your garlic as an odourless or reduced odour capsule. For severe headaches, you may want to supplement with as much as 1000 mg garlic oil capsules three times daily.

Periwinkle

This flower, commonly used for ground cover in hard-to-garden areas, was used by medieval healers to relieve the pain of headaches. Periwinkle contains a substance called vincamine which, according to medical research, appears to increase blood flow to the brain. One German study which used EEG readings to monitor changes in brain activity confirmed this and found that in addition to increased cerebral blood flow, vincamine also increased cerebral oxygen consumption, both of which will help to reduce headache pain. The researchers concluded that periwinkle had a generally tonifying effect on the blood vessels in the brain.

There are few cautions with this herb, although the experience of herbal practitioners is that people with low blood pressure should avoid using it. No texts give this warning, but vincamine is potentially hypotensive. Because of this, periwinkle is not available in all countries worldwide. In Europe you can still buy it and it is often an ingredient in herbal pain relief remedies. However, it is not available in America, where the Food and Drug Administration have expressed doubts about its use.

Valerian

Since a large number of headaches are associated with emotional anxiety, stress and lack of sleep, you should consider keeping some valerian in your herbal medicine chest. Valerian is one of the most potent herbal remedies for the relief of insomnia and has been shown to be at least as effective as benzodiazpines — but without the adverse effects. Valerian combines well with another sedative herb, passion flower, and many over-the-counter herbal remedies contain both.

No adverse effects have been observed with valerian. However, be mindful that you do not need to take large doses to produce good results. Indeed, studies show that the quality of sleep is not improved with larger doses. In one study, 900 mg of valerian extract was no more powerful than 450 mg. Since it is obviously a powerful sedative, it is always best to take the minimum amount you can to produce restful sleep.

CHAPTER 8

Homeopathy

Homeopathy is one of the most gentle and yet most powerful alternatives there is. It has never been shown to produce any adverse effects and an increasing number of people find it remarkably effective for the treatment of a wide range of disorders.

Homeopathic treatment is based on the principle that like cures like, or the 'similar principle'. Thus the patient will be given a remedy which under normal circumstances would produce the same symptoms which they are currently suffering from. This is in complete contrast to conventional medicine, which traditionally treats a patient's symptoms with medicines which have the opposite effect. So, for example, a patient suffering from constipation would be given something to loosen the bowels and someone suffering headache pain is given medicines which block the pain.

In homeopathy, infinitesimal doses of medicines derived from a variety of plant, mineral, chemical and animal sources are used. These minute doses are used to produce change and enhance the body's own capacity for both physical and emotional healing.

Homeopathy is a discipline which has been well researched and shown to work on a wide range of physical and emotional states. Homeopathy aims to treat the whole person, thus individually chosen homeopathic remedies may help treat both the physical and emotional states which can trigger persistent and chronic headaches. Although many people report a swift and profound relief from their symptoms with homeopathy, most studies show that homeopathy tends to work slowly but produces long-lasting results.

One of the reasons why it works so well for a large number of people is that treatment is based on the total symptom picture and the individual nature of the patient. Homeopathic evaluation is comprehensive and your practitioner will take a detailed personal history. Rather than just suppressing symptoms, a homeopath will aim to address the underlying cause. Because homeopathic remedies are safe and unlikely to produce side-effects, they are appropriate for all groups including the elderly and perhaps especially children.

Once the history taking is done, a homeopathic practitioner will study your pattern of symptoms and choose a remedy which is best for you. You can do the same thing, albeit on a rather more limited scale. Your headache diary will help you to identify your major symptoms. It is particularly important if you are a beginner or are self-diagnosing to stick to major symptom patterns as the key to choosing a remedy. Compare your symptoms to those indicated for each remedy and try the one which most closely matches your own pattern.

If you select the wrong remedy, it simply won't work and you will not suffer any unpleasant side-effects. It is important if you are self-diagnosing and buying homeopathic remedies over the counter not to use them as you would a conventional remedy. Often a single dose is all that is required. This is something which can be very difficult to take on board if you have spent years taking medicine on a three or four times daily schedule. If you are uncertain about how to take a remedy and the remedies label is unclear, it is best to consult a qualified therapist for advice.

Taking and Storing Homeopathic Remedies

Homeopathic remedies are available in a bafflingly wide range of doses from specialist suppliers. However, the remedies which you can buy in most health food shops are commonly sold in two strengths, 6c and 30c (though occasionally the c is omitted on the label). This is a centesimal dose, meaning that the remedy has been diluted one part remedy to ninety-nine parts water and alcohol. In a 6c remedy, for example, this process will have taken place six times. Less is more in homeopathy and although the 30c remedy has been diluted more times, it is considered more potent. Follow the dosage instruction on the label unless otherwise instructed. During a headache attack, try using one 6c tablet every half hour for occasional complaints, or one 30c tablet every half hour for more acute conditions. Stop taking the remedy at the first sign of improvement or after four hours, whichever comes first.

Homeopathic remedies are very delicate and certain things will act as an antidote to them. You should not take a remedy less than twenty minutes before or after food. Also avoid strong, highly flavoured foods and other items such as mints or cloves immediately before or after taking a remedy. While you are taking a homeopathic remedy, you should switch to a non-mint toothpaste — those flavoured with fennel are a particularly a good choice. You should not touch remedies with your bare hands. Always tip them straight from the lid of your storage bottle into your mouth. To make this easier, some commercially available remedies now come in single dose dispensers. Remedies should always be stored in a cool dark place.

Homeopathy for Headaches

Scientists who do not believe that infinitesimal doses can work conclude that homeopathic cures are all in the mind. To test this theory, they compare the effect of homeopathic remedies against placebos — inert substances which are not thought to cause any reaction in the body.

While studies into homeopathy have turned up mixed results, the general trend suggests that once the right remedy is selected the patient experiences a reduction in the frequency, duration and severity of headache pain. Mixed results in studies may be in part because researchers seldom allow for changing to a more suitable remedy should the first one fail to produce the desired results, as would happen in a genuine homeopathic consultation.

In one German study in 1991, which looked at eight different remedies (singly or in a combination of two) compared with a placebo, homeopathy significantly reduced the number of headaches from ten attacks per month to 1.8 per month at the end of four months. This compared favourably to those individuals who were given a placebo; they experienced a much smaller reduction, from 9.9 per month to 7.9 per month.

When researchers at the Princess Margaret Migraine Clinic in London undertook a four-month trial of homeopathy in 1997, both groups improved (homeopathy nineteen per cent, placebo sixteen per cent). Eleven different homeopathic remedies were used in all and at first this seemed a disappointing result. But closer scrutiny revealed that the placebo really only worked best on those suffering from mild migraine attacks, while homeopathy seemed most effective on moderate to severe attacks. Most importantly, improvement in the placebo group began to reverse itself after the fourth month, while slow improvement continued in the homeopathy group.

Which Remedy?

While almost any homeopathic remedy can help headache, some are more commonly used than others. If after looking at the ten most common remedies listed below you are still unsure which remedy is most suited to your symptom pattern, homeopath Dana Ullman recommends trying either *Belladonna*, *Bryonia* or *Nux vomica*, since these cover the most commonly experienced symptoms.

Belladonna

This remedy is indicated for those who are experiencing intense, violent throbbing or drumming pain. The *Belladonna* headache can cause extreme sensitivity and the least bit of light, noise, touch, strong or unusual smells, motion or jarring brings on a new wave of pain. The pain can begin suddenly and it may also go away suddenly. It may spread throughout the entire head or be localised in the forehead, from where it may extend to the back of the head. Often the pupils are dilated and the face is flushed or feels hot, or there may be a high fever. Sometimes the hands and feet are cold.

The *Belladonna* headache characteristically strikes in the afternoon. Often the pain is made worse by climbing stairs, as well as travelling down a slope, escalator or stairway. Hot sun will also aggravate the pain. Firm pressure to the head will often make the headache feel better, as will sitting down.

Bryonia

A *Bryonia* headache is also aggravated by motion. In fact, this is one of its most important features. Even slight motion of the eyes can make this headache worse. The pain can also be made worse by slight touch. It is generally worse in the morning and though it may be felt immediately upon waking, it is just as likely to come on only after the person first moves in bed or gets out of bed. The pain is generally located in the forehead and extends to the back of the head, but is commonly centred over the left eye. It is experienced as a steady ache with very little throbbing; sometimes there is a sense of fullness or heaviness in the head. During an attack, the head may also feel bruised. Nausea and vomiting and especially constipation may occur. You may feel irritable and irascible and want to be left alone.

This headache is better from firm pressure, rest, lying on the painful side and cool drinks or compresses.

Gelsemium

A good remedy for muscle contraction headaches. The pain is often right-sided and generally begins at the back of the head, often extending to the rest of the head or forehead. You may feel as though a band or hoop were bound tightly around your head. Or your head will feel full and swollen and your face can be purple and congested looking. You may also feel dull, aching and apathetic, with a weak, heavy feeling in your limbs. Your eyes may droop and you may look exhausted. *Gelsemium* is one of the few homeopathic remedies indicated for headaches preceded by a dimness of vision or the other visual disturbances so common in migraine attacks. The pain of this headache is not much affected by changes in room temperature, but other environmental factors such as light, noise, motion and jarring do aggravate it. Napping, damp weather, tobacco smoke and strong emotions will make the pain worse. Though not particularly irritable, you will feel like being left alone.

The pain is generally better for being in the open air, putting your head between your knees, movement and stimulants such as coffee.

Natrum Mur

This type of headache can be brought on by bright sunlight or by prolonged periods of coughing. The pain can be blinding and it may feel as if your head is bursting or being pounded by a thousand tiny hammers. It is generally worse in the top of the head or over the eyes. Your face may lose all its colour during an attack, which may last from sunrise to sunset.

Pain can be accompanied by feelings of depression and the need to be alone. Any kind of mental effort, noise or touch will tend to make the symptoms worse and you will not want to talk to or receive sympathy from others during an attack.

What makes the pain better is cool, fresh air, or a cool bath, resting with your head elevated, being left alone and skipping a meal.

Nux Vomica

Nux headaches are often brought on by overindulgence in something, either food, drink, drugs or staying up too late. They can make you feel as if you have been beaten about the head. These headaches are generally accompanied by irritability and a general feeling of sickness and digestive upsets. You may have a bitter or sour taste in your mouth in the morning and queasiness, dizziness, nausea or vomiting (dry heaves and gas are typical symptoms). The pain can be brought on by long periods of concentrated mental work and cold air and wind will make it worse.

This headache tends to be more prominent in the morning, particularly upon first waking, and tends to get better after the person is up and about. As with most headaches, motion may aggravate symptoms, but shaking the head will be particularly painful. Lying on the painful side often makes the pain worse, and the sound of footsteps may be particularly irritating to you.

Wrapping the head or being in a warm room may help to relieve the pain.

Phosphorous

This is a good remedy to choose if your headaches are brought on by changes in atmospheric conditions, for example before a thunder storm. It can also be brought on by hunger, fright or a shock. The pain of a *Phosphorous* headache usually manifests as an aching over one eye. It is generally a throbbing, burning pain and can be accompanied by dizziness and vertigo. Being touched and lying on the painful side will make it worse, as will cold air and mental effort. These headaches tend to be worse in the morning and evening.

Lying in a darkened room, massage, eating, a cool shower or bath and a nap will often help improve symptoms.

Pulsatilla

These headaches often come on after meals, particularly if you have been eating warm, rich or fatty foods or ice-cream. Nausea, digestive upset and vomiting may also be a feature. Pulsatilla is good for those headaches which coincide with the menstrual cycle — before, during and especially when the period ends — and also those that result from a frightening experience. The throbbing pain is most often felt in the forehead or on one side; however, it may change location frequently. Walking briskly may make the pain worse, whereas gentle motion, especially walking about slowly in the open air, may make the pain better. Pressure will also relieve the pain, but blowing the nose aggravates it.

The *Pulsatilla* individual is emotionally mild and sensitive and may be moved to weep from the pain. Though a little irritable, the person is likely to want company and consolation.

Sanguinaria

Typically, this headache begins in the back of the head, but extends to and soon settles over the right eye or in the right side of the head. Right-sided headaches are covered by other remedies such as *Gelsemium*, but *Sanguinaria* is especially noted for this symptom. The pain is sharp, splitting, knife-like and sometimes throbbing. Once again, nausea and vomiting occur at the height of the pain. Vomiting in particular may provide relief from the pain. Motion will make the pain worse, whereas sleep and firm pressure relieve it.

This remedy suits headaches which occur in a consistent pattern, such as every seven days, and may be useful for cluster headaches or if you are having a classic migraine with visual-aura symptoms.

Sepia

Sepia headaches are usually connected with digestive symptoms. Often they are brought on by skipping a meal. This headache can produce stinging, shooting pains over one eye — usually the left — accompanied by nausea and dizziness. In some cases, the roots of your hair will feel sensitive. The pain tends to strike in the late afternoons and evenings and is made worse by damp atmospheres, just before your period, from bending over and from sex. You may also feel depressed and unable to cope.

Vigorous exercise in the fresh air can make the headache better, as will pressure and warm compresses on the painful points.

Sulphur

This is another headache which can be caused by low blood sugar. *Sulphur* types need to eat small regular meals to combat hypoglycaemia. The pain is somewhat different from *Sepia*, in that it is best described as a sick headache. You may feel dizzy and there will be a heavy, throbbing sensation in the crown of the head, or a feeling as if your brain was being squeezed. There may be pressure in the temples. This type of headache is made worse by becoming over-heated, especially in bed, and by exertion. Alcohol will also make it worse. It tends to strike in the mid-morning and can also be brought on by consuming sweet foods.

Fresh air, particularly if the weather is warm and dry, movement and walking all help to alleviate the pain.

CHAPTER 9

Acupuncture

Holistic practitioners and medical scientists agree on one thing: all life is made of energy. According to the Chinese, the life energy which surrounds and flows through us is called Qi, or Ch'i (pronounced *chee*). When this life force is disturbed, either because it is blocked or because it is moving too slow or too fast, imbalance and eventually illness will result. The Chinese believe that headaches are the result of blood stagnation and that stimulation of specific acupuncture points can help to relieve this stagnation.

The word acupuncture has two roots in Latin: *acus* meaning needle and *punctura*, to puncture. In China thousands of years ago, a strange war-time phenomenon was observed. Soldiers whose bodies were pierced by arrows sometimes recovered from illnesses which had plagued them for many years. Eventually the idea evolved that, by penetrating the skin at certain points, diseases could be cured.

Although acupuncture has been an important part of traditional Chinese medicine for more than 2500 years, it is only over the last twenty years or so that it has come to be more widely accepted by healthcare practitioners and the general public. The World Health Organization (WHO) has gone so far as to state that there is now sufficient medical evidence to support the effectiveness of acupuncture for it to be considered as an important part of primary health care. Perhaps as a result, the usually conservative medical press is devoting more and more space to acupuncture. Recently, the *Journal of the American Medical Association* devoted an entire issue to alternative health-care. In it was a strong validation of acupuncture. The WHO has gone even further by recommending that acupuncture should be fully integrated into conventional medicine. Strong words, but then acupuncture can be strong medicine.

There are over 2000 acupuncture points on the body. These run along twelve meridians, or energy channels. Each meridian is a biological pathway linked to a particular organ in the body; thus each organ can be treated by stimulating the relevant meridian. In everyday practice, only about 200 acupuncture points are commonly used. These are stimulated by fine needles which unblock the flow of Qi at these points. Your practitioner may use his fingers to manipulate the needles; or he may opt to use electroacupuncture, in which a small amount of electricity is passed through the needles in order to simulate a particular point.

The flow of life energy can be disturbed by many things, including illness and emotional states. Using needles as fine as a human hair, your acupuncturist will aim to activate your body's energy channels, to treat disease, boost your immune system, promote your body's natural healing powers and alleviate fatigue. Because it is safe and effective, with no known side-effects, even those who feel a little nervous about the idea of needles find acupuncture an effective option.

Acupuncture has been shown to ease disturbances of the digestive, hormonal and circulatory systems. For some people, it has provided relief from structural problems and painful inflammatory problems such as arthritis, trauma and back pain — all causes of recurrent head pain.

In addition to treating specific problems, another bonus of acupuncture is that it may help to strengthen the body generally. It can help to stimulate the immune system and has a beneficial effect on the circulation, blood pressure, the rhythm of the heart and the secretion of gastric juices. It may also stimulate a variety of hormones which help the body respond more efficiently to injury and stress.

Acupuncture for Headaches

Acupuncture can affect a cure over the longer term by treating underlying imbalances in the body, but it also has a short-term effect. Many patients find swift relief from symptoms after a session of acupuncture, since the needles, when properly placed, seem to activate the body's own pain-killing chemicals. This is one reason why acupuncture has been used successfully in patients undergoing surgery and also to reduce the pain of giving birth.

The precise mechanism by which acupuncture works to relieve headaches is not entirely clear. It does not appear to increase levels of endorphins — the body's natural pain killers. Levels of these may be low in migraine sufferers anyway, and studies which have aimed to assess whether acupuncture can raise endorphin levels have not been successful. What acupuncture appears to do is increase levels of another chemical called serotonin — which enhances our feelings of well-being and also regulates the diameter of blood vessels.

Studies into acupuncture for headaches have been encouraging. For instance, over eight months, one small study in New Zealand of people who had experienced severe, regular migraine for more than five years showed positive results. In it, acupuncture was compared to a placebo as well as to the opioid analgesic, naloxone. Acupuncture was found to have the most significant effect, with forty per cent of subjects showing a fifty to one hundred per cent reduction in the number of headaches and their duration. Although pain sensation was not altered, attacks were less severe and less often accompanied by nausea and vomiting.

Another study concluded that electroacupuncture was most effective in treating muscle contraction headaches. Of 177 patients with long-term, chronic head and face pain, acupuncture reduced pain in one hundred (fifty-six per cent) of the group. Two years later, researchers found that forty-seven per cent of those who had improved had elected to carry on with the treatment on a long-term basis, and were experiencing periods of relief of up to two years. Moreover, twenty-one per cent had discontinued treatment on the basis of complete and prolonged relief from pain.

In a study comparing acupuncture to the beta-blocker drug metoprolol, acupuncture was shown to be at least as effective in reducing the frequency and duration of attacks (though not their severity), and superior in terms of negative side-effects. Other studies comparing acupuncture with conventional treatment have found similar results.

Acupressure

If you are still not convinced, or simply don't like the idea of needles, acupressure, which works on the same points but using finger pressure instead of needles, can also be helpful for most headache types. Unlike acupuncture, acupressure does not need to be applied by a professional — simple acupressure techniques can be learned by anyone. Those who follow this discipline believe that pain almost anywhere in the body can be relieved within minutes by using the oriental self-help technique called G-jo acupressure.

G-jo means first aid in Chinese. There are at least twenty important acupoints for relieving the many types of headaches that Western medicine has identified. Fortunately, you do not need to learn them all, since there are several broadly acting points on the body which can produce immediate, often miraculous, results.

Two points are particularly useful for headaches:

1. G-jo 13, which is in the webbing between the thumb and
    forefinger. To find it, squeeze the two together, place a
    finger atop the fleshy mound that is formed. Keep your
    finger on the mound and relax your hand. Then begin to
    stimulate the point, first with deep pressure and after a few
    seconds with a kind of digging massage. The more this place
    hurts, the more it is likely to be the right place for you to
    stimulate during a headache. Avoid stimulating this point
    during pregnancy.

2. G-jo 4 is located on the arm in line with the middle finger.
    To find it, bend your wrist backwards and measure two
    thumb widths above the most prominent crease in your
    upper wrist. You should feel a slight hollow in between the
    two bones of the arm. Relax your wrist, find the tender
    spot and stimulate it in the same way as G-jo 13 for a few
    seconds.

When stimulating these two points, you may have to press for
a minute or so (no more). Once you have done one side, then
do the other. Always release the pressure when a change occurs
in your symptoms; your body will then take over the healing
process.

Occasionally you may experience minor reactions when
applying these simple, self-help techniques. These can include a
slight flush or perspiration across the brow or shoulders; indeed
you may feel warmth and clamminess anywhere on the body.
These are normal reactions and pass quickly. Most people report
a profound sense of relief after stimulating the right acupoint.

CHAPTER 10

Hypnotherapy

The power of suggestion can be powerful medicine. Hypnotherapy uses this power to induce a trance-like state that enables an individual to explore the deepest levels of their mind, body and emotions. While in a trance, positive suggestions can then be made and heard at a very deep level in the patient to help bring about change. Hypnotherapy is so effective that it has been used by dentists and doctors in lieu of an anaesthetic. There is even a case of a fifteen-year-old girl undergoing a heart operation while under hypnosis.

Hypnosis is one of the oldest forms of therapy. Ancient writings confirm that the Sumerians used hypnosis as a therapeutic tool. Specially trained healers gave sufferers hypnotic suggestions, as did the later Hindu fakirs, the Persian magi and the Indian yogi. The Ebers papyrus tells us that ancient Egyptian priest-doctors would ask sufferers to fix their gaze upon a glossy piece of metal to help induce a trance-like state. It's a technique which is still commonly used by modern practitioners.

Today, the vast majority, as many as ninety-four per cent of patients, derive some benefit from hypnotherapy. Relaxation is the most commonly reported effect, but it has been used to treat a wide range of conditions including headache, respiratory problems, sleep disorders, stress and chronic pain.

The mind is divided into two parts, the conscious and unconscious. Some practitioners liken it to an iceberg: the conscious mind is the tip, the unconscious is the large mass which lies beneath the surface. What lurks in the unconscious is often at the root of our health problems, since body and mind are constantly interacting in ways which the conscious mind is not aware of.

In order to function on a day-to-day basis, we need to remain on a conscious level. But this does not mean that we should avoid the unconscious. A number of people find the idea of confronting the unconscious frightening — almost like having to walk down a dark, unfamiliar street in the dead of night. But the unconscious isn't just a chaotic jumble of scary memories and dark secrets. It also holds all of our potential for good, as well as our under-used creative talents and our richest emotions. For many people, hypnotherapy is a way to access the good as well as the unfamiliar and scary. It is a way to address these things in a safe, controlled way.

Hypnosis is not the same as sleep. When the brain waves of hypnotised subjects have been monitored, what has been revealed is an increase in alpha wave activity. These are the electrical impulses which are produced when humans are in a relaxed but mentally alert state. When a person is asleep, slower delta waves are the predominant type of brain activity. Given this, it's perhaps not surprising that the overwhelming experience of hypnotherapy patients is one of relaxation and relief.

For hypnosis to work, you must have the desire to be hypnotised. Your willingness to take this step is what opens the door to a dialogue with your unconscious self. People who have lived with headache pain for years often forget what it is like to live without pain. The pain becomes deeply ingrained as part of their personality. They may even believe, on some level, that they need pain in order to make them feel alive. One benefit of hypnosis is that it can take you back to a time when you were generally pain free and help you to re-experience what that was like. It can provide positive, supportive suggestions which can help you create new, pain-free patterns in your life. For instance, if your headache is a response to stress, you can begin to build new, more positive responses to help you deal with stress.

Hypnotherapy for Headaches

Hypnotherapy has increasingly been the focus of research trials and there is now a good deal of evidence to suggest that hypnosis, though it works primarily on the mind, produces a number of profound physical effects. These include a slower heartbeat and breathing rate, dilation of the bronchi in the lungs, lowered blood pressure, and more efficient production of stomach acid.

It is also thought that hypnotherapy can produce a positive change in immune system function, making it an ideal tool for treating a range of health disorders, such as tension headaches and other stress-related problems.

Hypnotherapy can be performed with a practitioner, or the method can be taught to individuals who can then practise self-hypnosis as either a preventative or cure. It is particularly useful for headaches which stem from stress, anxiety and depression. For instance, when researchers from Brigham and Women's Hospital in Boston, Massachusetts used hypnotherapy to ease chronic tension headaches among patients, they discovered that the duration of the headache and its intensity were significantly reduced by the therapy. In another study, hypnotherapy was shown to be more than three times more effective at producing complete remission of symptoms of migraine than the conventional drug prochlorperazine (Stemetil).

A comparison of self-hypnosis with the drug propranolol in children aged six to twelve years with classic migraine, who had had no previous specific treatment, showed that while self-hypnosis did not alter the severity of attacks, it did reduce the number of attacks the children had.

Studies into hypnotherapy prove that mind and body are intimately connected. In one study, researchers in the Netherlands compared autogenic training (a form of relaxation therapy) to self-hypnosis and found no differences between the two techniques. However they did find a clue to why some patients improve and others do not. Seeking out an alternative therapy often represents a commitment to yourself and your own well-being. In this study, those who perceived pain relief as a result of their own efforts (i.e. to acknowledge the need for help and seek appropriate treatment, in this case learning and applying self-hypnosis) experienced longer-term relief.

Later, some of the researchers from this same group went on to study whether it was possible to predict who would experience pain reduction through hypnosis by studying outside factors such as the health status of the patient and their psychological profile. What they found was that those who were confident of a cure at the pre-treatment stage achieved greater pain reduction — a phenomenon not unknown in other areas of medicine.

Self-Hypnosis

If you are seeing a hypnotherapist, the chances are that he or she will give you some self-hypnosis suggestions which you can practise at home. These usually involve taking a few moments each day to relax and reinforce the positive suggestions which you will have received during your formal session.

Anyone can practise simple self-hypnosis at any time. You will need to be somewhere quiet where you can be assured of few distractions. You should be sitting comfortably in a chair. You should also be clear about what you would like to achieve, for example complete relaxation of your tense muscles, letting go of obsessive thoughts or steadying your nerves.

Begin by focusing on a point in front of you. It can be anything — a picture, a pattern on the wallpaper, a place where the light is reflected on the wall. Let everything except that object drop away from your mind. Stare at the object until you begin to see it change. That's the signal to close your eyes. Now let your attention come to your body. Pick somewhere in your body that you are particularly aware of at that moment. It could be your eyelids or the way your lungs are taking in air, it could even be your aching head. Let everything else drop away and focus on this point in your body until you feel a change: your breathing may slow down, or a tense muscle may begin to relax.

Once you reach this stage, you can help yourself go into a deeper trance by counting backwards from ten to zero. Some people like to imagine that they are descending a staircase and that with each step they are becoming more relaxed and receptive. Using the opposite method, counting up and ascending the staircase, is a good gentle way of coming out of hypnosis.

When you are in this trance-like state, find as many different ways of saying the same positive things to yourself as you can. It may help to write out beforehand a few statements you can use during self-hypnosis. Try to keep these positive; instead of saying 'I will not be tense' say 'I am relaxed and calm.' Or instead of saying 'I won't let the pressure get on top of me' say 'I am coping well with all the things I have to do.'

Try also to make good use of your imagination. If you are tense about something you have to do at work, imagine yourself coping well and with confidence at each stage of the day: getting up, travelling to work, arriving at work, seeing your colleagues, taking meetings, and so on. Let yourself explore all the possibilities of the day, and your reactions to them, reminding yourself at each stage that you are coping in a relaxed and positive way.

Remember that negative patterns take a long time to build up and they can take an equally long time to knock down. Just doing this type of exercise once or twice is unlikely to produce great results. You will need to practise each day for a month or more even to begin to feel a change occurring in yourself and in the way you respond to outside forces. Like many alternative therapies, hypnotherapy requires a commitment to yourself and your own well-being. It also requires a commitment of time in order to restructure the less positive aspects of your personality and to bring out your best qualities.

CHAPTER 11

Osteopathy and Chiropractic

When headaches are the result of neck injury or strain, osteopathy or chiropractic intervention is often of great benefit. Osteopathy and chiropractic evolved around the same time and largely along the same lines. Both osteopaths and chiropractors believe that subtle and not-so-subtle misalignments of the body can result in illness. Because of this, people who consult either type of practitioner often come to rely on them to treat a whole range of health problems.

Osteopathy

Osteopathy is a distinct system of diagnosis and treatment which can be used on its own or in conjunction with conventional treatments. It is a hands-on therapy, where the practitioner is concerned with the interrelationship between the structure of the body (in other words, the muscles and skeletal system) and the way in which the body functions.

However, many osteopaths see their roles as encompassing more than just fixing mechanical dysfunctions. Many osteopaths are interested not only in the structure of the spine, but the subtle movement of energy through the body and how it affects mind, body and emotions. Therefore some practitioners will undertake the treatment of respiratory, gastrointestinal and cardiovascular problems by aiming to restore the free flow of vital energy to these areas.

86

Others believe osteopathy to be an effective treatment for stress, anxiety and depression. In addition, some osteopaths are trained in a combination of osteopathy and naturopathy and will approach their practice from a more holistic, naturopathic point of view. Clearly, the way one osteopath works may be very different from the way another works, so it is important to discuss what conditions your practitioner feels comfortable with treating before you begin.

Osteopaths work with their hands, using a variety of treatments. These may include gentle pressure on the soft tissues or scalp. The latter technique is called cranial osteopathy and is particularly suitable to young children. Some will use rhythmic movement and occasionally more forceful techniques to mobilise stiff joints.

Chiropractic

Chiropractic developed around the same time as osteopathy and is used to treat the same kinds of musculoskeletal problems. Nevertheless, there are subtle differences in the approach which chiropractors take. Chiropractic concerns itself mostly with the spinal column and the effects of misalignments of the spinal joints. Chiropractors believe that misalignment of these joints can result in poor health, especially in the nervous system and the organs of the body.

In chiropractic, the spinal column is of supreme importance, since it acts as a kind of switchboard for the rest of the body. If bones move out of place due to soft tissue damage, allergies, sensitivities, tension or toxic build-up, the nerve interference caused can result in chronic illness and pain such as headaches, digestive disturbances, PMS and emotional problems.

While a great many patients report tremendous success with both osteopathy and chiropractic in treating a wide range of disorders, osteopathy has not benefited from the same scientific attention as chiropractic. This is in part because in the

US a chiropractor must also be a fully qualified doctor. This has elevated chiropractic in the eyes of the medical establishment and enabled funding for observational research.

Chiropractic is a more commonly used therapy in the US, where there are over 55,000 practitioners treating an estimated 15 to 20 million patients each year. In the UK, osteopathy is the more popular therapy and it is practised by specially trained non-physicians.

Hands-on Therapy for Headaches

Tension headaches can particularly benefit from treatment by an osteopath or chiropractor. In America, the National Institutes of Health have concluded that chiropractic manipulation is better than drugs for the long-term management of chronic headaches. Chiropractic research, for instance, estimates that once the cause of the headache is identified, around eighty per cent of those treated can experience long-term benefits after just a few short sessions.

Both types of practitioner will take a full history from you and discuss with you the nature of your headache. They may ask you questions about whether you sit for prolonged periods at work or at home, check your posture and ask about previous injuries which may have involved the head, neck, spine or joints.

If your headache has a structural or postural root, the chiropractor or osteopath can help realign your body and release tension. If the structural problem is caused by something other than soft tissue damage, your practitioner may recommend that you follow a complementary regime to maintain your health. This may involve altering your diet or using herbs to flush toxins out of your system and improve immune system function.

There is an astonishing, and not altogether logical, reluctance on the part of conventional medicine to admit that spinal manipulation can help relieve headaches. Even those who find positive results are often reluctant to shout about them. For instance, one major American analysis of chiropractic research from 1966 to the present day aimed to assess just how effective the therapy was in the treatment of neck pain and headache. The researchers scanned four computerised databases and retrieved 134 studies for analysis. After a review of the evidence, which showed that at the very least spinal manipulation provided short-term benefits for some, had only a small complication rate and compared favourably with the use of muscle relaxants, the authors only grudgingly concluded that chiropractic 'may' be of use in some cases.

The benefits of spinal manipulation over conventional drug treatments have been seen in other studies. In another US study, a group of 150 subjects with chronic tension headaches were randomly assigned to receive either 10-30 mg of the anti-depressant/ sedative amitriptyline at bedtime for six weeks, or chiropractic treatment twice weekly for six weeks. Results showed that while both groups improved at similar rates at first, a follow-up consultation four weeks after the treatment ceased showed that only the chiropractic group were experiencing continued relief from their headache pain.

In this study, more than eighty per cent of the drug group reported side-effects such as drowsiness, dry mouth and weight gain, as opposed to around four per cent in the manipulation group who reported neck soreness and stiffness as the main side-effects. Again, the conclusion was somewhat grudging. The authors suggested that because of small numbers, the study was not conclusive and that further studies should control for the placebo effect (in other words, the ability of a placebo to pro-vide a cure for some people) of the doctor-patient relationship. One wonders when medical research will also control for the nocebo effect (the ability of a doctor's attitude, personality and beliefs to negatively influence their patient's health) of the doctor-patient relationship!

Perhaps one of the biggest benefits of spinal manipulation is that it can help reduce your intake of pain killers. Since the overuse of these has been associated with a number of health problems, including stomach upsets and rebound headaches, this is a real plus. In one small study of patients suffering from chronic headache, half received spinal manipulation twice weekly and the other half received laser treatment combined with deep friction massage twice a week for three weeks.

Researchers found that while the use of pain killers decreased by thirty-six per cent in the spinal manipulation group, it remained unchanged in the massage group. The number of headaches per day also decreased, by sixty-nine per cent in the manipulation group compared with only thirty-six per cent in the massage group. Headache intensity also decreased by thirty-six per cent in the spinal manipulation group compared with a seventeen per cent decrease in the massage group.

If you are seeking out osteopathic or chiropractic help, you will probably get the best results if you combine this with self-help. For instance, it is no good having your spine realigned if you are just going to go back to sitting in the same unsupportive, uncomfortable chair or sleeping on the same sagging mattress day after day, or if you continue to adopt a posture which throws your spine and joints right back out again.

If your diet is inadequate or poor, it may be contributing to chronic musculoskeletal problems. Regimes such as Alexander Technique are particularly good in helping postural problems, and regular yoga will help keep your joints flexible. Without this kind of commitment to yourself, osteopathy and chiropractic may only be able to provide a band-aid therapy. As with any alternative therapy, there is an onus on the patient to make lifestyle changes to support the return to good health.

CHAPTER 12

Aromatherapy

Throughout history, volatile oils extracted from flowers, herbs and animal sources have been used to calm or stimulate the emotions and enhance well-being. Our sense of smell is the sense most directly linked to the emotional centres of the brain; pleasing smells can lift moods and have been known to alleviate certain symptoms, such as headache pain.

There are about 150 essential oils which are distilled from plants, flowers, trees, bark, grasses and seeds; each has a distinctive therapeutic, psychological and physiological effect. Some are antiseptic, others are anti-viral, anti-inflammatory, pain-relieving, antidepressant and expectorant. They can be used to stimulate, relax, improve digestion and eliminate excess water.

Essential oils should always be from natural sources. This is not mere snobbery, because if perfume was once an art, it is now strictly a science. The cosmetic industry long ago abandoned the use of genuinely natural ingredients. Today, it bases its products on fragrances derived from petrochemicals. These fragrances are used in cosmetics and household products as well as in foods, where they are called flavours or aromas. Flavours and aromas are also used heavily in the tobacco industry to enhance the flavour of cigarettes, especially the lower tar and nicotine brands.

Synthetic oils do not work in the same way as natural ones and may produce a range of undesired effects. Numerous bath preparations in particular say they contain 'natural' ingredients such as citrus or lavender. What they really mean is that they contain chemical fragrances which approximate the smell of these natural substances.

Studies have shown that inhaling synthetic fragrance chemicals can cause negative circulatory changes in the brain. Subtle negative changes in electrical activity in the brain can also occur with exposure to petrochemical fragrances. Perhaps not surprisingly, these types of fragrances are a frequent trigger of migraine headaches. When you are buying a fragrant oil, always make sure that the manufacturer has put the Latin name on the label; otherwise, you could be buying a synthetic oil or a mixture of oils derived from nature and synthetic oils made from petrochemicals.

Aromatherapy is suitable for self-help and is widely used in homes, clinics and hospitals for a variety of applications. They can be used in baths or steam inhalations, sprinkled on pillows or sheets, used in oil burners, diffusers and vaporisers. When aromatherapy is combined with massage it can have a profound effect on an individual's sense of well-being. Massage with essential oils is not only pleasant, it can help boost immunity — thus reducing the risk of contracting viral infections associated with headache.

Massage also has a psychological effect. Therapeutic touch has long been good medicine for those suffering from anxiety and depression.

Aromatherapy for Headaches

Different oils work in different ways. Most work indirectly to relieve pain; lavender oil, for instance, can be used to produce relaxation and promote sleep. But one oil, peppermint, has been shown to work directly to relieve pain. It is thought that peppermint oil possesses analgesic properties and works in part by stimulating the nerve fibres which register cold. This in turn reduces the pain information transmitted to the brain.

In trials with headache sufferers, peppermint has been combined with other, similar oils such as eucalyptus to gauge which combination is most effective in the treatment of headaches. The most effective combinations were those where peppermint was the dominant oil. For instance, while equal amounts of peppermint and eucalyptus increased subjects' mental agility and had a muscle- and mind-relaxing effect, peppermint with just traces of eucalyptus was shown to have a more significant analgesic effect, which contributed to reducing the pain of a tension headache.

While peppermint is a good first choice for the direct treatment of headache pain, some headaches respond to a more subtle approach, using more complex blends of oils. The beauty of aromatherapy is that you can take part in the process of healing by selecting and blending your own oils. With a few exceptions, such as tea tree and lavender, most essential oils are simply too strong to be used neat. Therefore, always mix your oils in a base or carrier oil before you apply them to your skin or put them into your bath. Any vegetable-based oil will do as a carrier, but many people prefer lighter oils such as sweet almond, apricot kernel or grapeseed oil.

You can use the following table to guide you in making up your own individual blends:

AMOUNT OF ESSENTIAL OIL	AMOUNT OF BASE OIL
1 drop	1 ml
2–5 drops	5 ml (approx 1 tsp)
4–10 drops	10 ml (approx 1 dessertspoon)
6–15 drops	15 ml (approx ½ oz or 1 tblsp)
8–20 drops	20 ml
10–25 drops	25 ml
12–30	30 ml (approx 1 oz)

Now, consider some of the following suggestions for pleasant relief from different sources of headache pain.

Insomnia

Since anxiety, stress and lack of sleep are often linked to chronic headaches, anything which reduces these triggers should also act to reduce the frequency of headaches. It is certainly worth considering using aromatherapy to help you sleep. Instead of taking sleeping pills, try altering the atmosphere of your room with the scent of lavender.

In one study from 1995 of patients suffering from long-term insomnia, sedatives were withdrawn and in their place lavender oil was used as an 'ambient odour' (in other words a diffuser was used to scent the air with lavender). Not only did the patients report getting more sleep, they reported better sleep. Lavender oil was shown to be as effective as medication, without any of the unpleasant side-effects. What is more, lavender oil helped reduce the restless, unrefreshing sleep which sometimes comes as a result of insomnia.

During the day, try mixing lavender with uplifting oils such as geranium, clary sage, lemon, neroli and Roman camomile.

Stress and Anxiety

In her famous book *The Fragrant Mind*, internationally renowned aromatherapist Valerie Ann Worwood suggests that all stress is not equal. In order to find relief from anxiety and stress, you will need to dig a little deeper and identify your individual responses to stress. Once identified, you can try any of these combinations to help ease the tension. These essential oils combinations should be mixed in approximately 30 ml (1 oz) of base oil.

For **tense** anxiety with symptoms of bodily tension and muscle aches and pain try mixing 10 drops of clary sage, 15 drops of lavender and 5 drops of Roman camomile.

For **restless** anxiety with symptoms such as dizziness, sweating, over-activity, heart palpitations, a lump in the throat and stomach upsets, try 5 drops of vetivier, 10 drops of juniper and 15 drops of cedarwood.

For **apprehensive** anxiety with symptoms including worrying, brooding, unease and a sense of foreboding, even paranoia, use 15 drops of bergamot, 5 drops of lavender and 10 drops of geranium.

Finally, for **repressed** anxiety with symptoms of edginess, lack of concentration, irritability, insomnia or chronic exhaustion, use 10 drops each of neroli, rose Otto and bergamot.

Any of these mixtures can be used in massage, put into the bath, inhaled with steam or put onto a warm or cool compress and applied to the head.

Depression

Many of the oils used for anxiety and stress are also effective for depression. However, for quick relief from a minor depressive state, citrus oils have been shown to be most effective. Try using mandarin, grapefruit, lemon or orange according to your inclination. These can be used in an oil burner to alter the atmosphere of your room or in a relaxing massage. If either of these methods is not practical, for instance if you are travelling or at work, sprinkle some citrus essential oil on a cotton handkerchief and carry it with you in a small plastic bag. When you feel your spirits flag, you can discreetly take the hankie out and inhale deeply two or three times for a refreshing boost.

Sinusitis

A combination of eucalyptus and menthol in an ointment has been shown to be effective in treating the symptoms of most upper respiratory tract infections. Both oils encourage the secretion of mucous and act as anti-microbials. If you cannot find a ready-made ointment, you can mix these in a carrier oil and apply around the nose or make a steam inhalation. Other helpful oils for sinusitis include lavender, tea tree, eucalyptus, rosemary, juniper, bergamot, hyssop, cajuput, niaouli, thyme and lemon oils, singly or in combination.

Try Tiger Balm

Although not strictly an essential oil, Tiger Balm contains a combination of essential oils which can provide quick first aid for headaches. You can purchase Tiger Balm (either the red or white formula — there is little difference, though enthusiasts swear that the red, with its addition of cinnamon oil, is stronger) in most chemist and health food shops. This is a surprisingly effective type of aromatherapy, which can be applied directly to the temples to ease tension headaches.

Tiger Balm contains several essential oils such as camphor, menthol, cajuput and clove oil, which have been shown to be effective in relieving muscular strain. They also act as vaso-dilators, ensuring an even flow of blood through the veins.

In one small but interesting Australian study, sufferers of tension headaches were given either Tiger Balm, a neutral oint-ment which had an added odour to give it a strong smell, or the headache medication acetaminophen. Sufferers were asked to record any changes in their headache pain over the course of three hours after administration of their treatment. Those using Tiger Balm reported a much greater improvement in their headaches within five minutes to two hours of using the treat-ment than those using the neutral ointment.

What is really interesting, however, is that after three hours there was no difference in the level of reduction of pain between the Tiger Balm users and those who took acetaminophen. In fact Tiger Balm delivered quicker relief, within five to fifteen minutes of using it. So Tiger Balm was better in the short term and equal to conventional drugs after three hours — and has no side-effects. Given this, which would you rather take?

CHAPTER 13

Children's Headaches

While children's headaches have the same root causes as those experienced by adults, their treatment may require a little more sensitivity. A child with a limited vocabulary may be unable to describe how his or her head feels. Ask most young children where it hurts and they are likely to point to their tummies — and indeed migraines in young children may be felt in the abdomen. While the vast majority of children's headaches can be safely treated at home or with the help of alternative therapies, parents may need to listen very carefully to diagnose the cause and thus the appropriate treatment for their child.

Like adults, children's headaches generally follow a pattern, though there are some differences in the type of headache and their patterns as experienced by children. One reason for this is that children suffer from a different range of illnesses to adults. Children are unlikely to have neck injuries, although osteopaths would argue that obstetrically managed birth, which is not generally gentle birth, often constitutes a trauma to the neck and head. They will not be suffering from menstrual difficulties, strokes or high blood pressure. Children will, however, have more fevers and a wider range of completely new viral and bacterial infections which their immature immune systems must learn to deal with; they may have more eye and tooth problems as well.

For children, the world, which is full of teachers, bullies, marital disharmony, sibling rivalry, and TV and videos which present a very frightening view of life, is more emotionally challenging.

Perhaps not surprisingly, many children experience their first headaches around the age of four — just about the time they first enter school. School age is potentially emotionally upsetting and exhausting — many children are in school and play centres for longer than most adults work. It is also the time when children, under pressure from their peers, begin eating more junk such as chocolate, crisps and sugary drinks. This is also when sports and extra-curricular activities become more common. But even fun activities can be overdone and cause fatigue, and not surprisingly the most common type of headache children get is the tension headache.

Young children can also suffer from migraines, but again the pattern is somewhat different than for adults. While adult migraine is more common in women, in children under twelve migraine is more common in boys. It is only from puberty that the trend once again shifts in favour of females. Both types of headache can be disruptive in a child's life and children suffering from headaches lose more than twice the number of school days than children who do not.

Take It Seriously

Often children complaining of headache are not given the consideration they deserve. In one Finnish study of nearly 1000 children around the age of seven, around twenty per cent of children experienced headaches severe enough to disrupt their daily activities at least once in their lives. Less than a quarter of these children had been taken to a doctor to investigate the headache and only a small percentage of those children with migraine had been diagnosed before the study.

POTENTIALLY DANGEROUS HEADACHES

Though rare, headaches can sometimes be symptoms of a serious problem such as meningitis. You should call a doctor if your child's headache:

◆ Is accompanied by fever, vomiting, stiff neck, lethargy or confusion

◆ Follows a head injury

◆ Occurs in the morning accompanied by nausea

◆ Increases in severity over the course of a day or from one day to the next

◆ Is suddenly brought on by a sneeze or a cough

◆ Interferes with school or other activities

◆ Is restricted to one side of the head.

This study yielded some interesting information about the causes of children's headaches. For example, most started in the afternoon and were made worse by physical activity. The researchers also found that children who have headaches were more likely to grind their teeth at night and thus report tenderness around the jaw and in the neck muscles.

Whatever the cause, children's headaches should always be taken seriously. Not because they are a sign that something is seriously wrong — this is rarely the case — but because children are much less adept at handling pain than adults. They don't rationalise it away; all they know is that it hurts and they want somebody or something to make it better.

Try These First

It is particularly important with children to avoid the trap of providing a pill for every pain. This introduces a very poor attitude to health and illness at a young and vulnerable age. Instead, try some of the following suggestions:

Quiet things down. Try not to load your child's schedule up with lots of activities — however convenient it may be for you. Instead, every day should have a time when your child can paint or play quietly. Better still, use this time to play quietly or read with your child.

Talk to your child. If the headache seems to be in response to emotional tension, try to discover the source of the tension and deal with it. Just letting your child know you care is good medicine, since sometimes tension headaches are cries for attention.

Give your child some sense of control over their day-to-day lives. Children, like adults, are more prone to headaches when they feel out of control and pushed around. If your child is stressed out or has a problem, don't try to 'fix' it for them. Instead, encourage a dialogue where your child can come up with his or her own unique solutions.

Rub it away. If the muscles around the temples are tender, gently rubbing them can bring relief. If they are too tender and your child says stop, then stop. But many children simply like being touched and stroked gently by their parents. If your child gets a headache in his or her tummy, try rubbing the abdomen gently in a clockwise direction. Children also respond well to foot massage.

Keep their blood sugar up with sensible foods. Make sure breakfasts are nourishing and that lunches actually get eaten instead of traded away or thrown in the bin. Skipping a meal can bring on a headache or make an existing one worse in some children.

Cut out caffeine. Your child's headache could be a rebound headache caused by the caffeine in sodas and chocolates. These are empty foods anyway and should be restricted to an occasional treat.

Use the G-jo acupressure technique recommended on page 80.

Persistent headache. If the headache persists, have your child lie down in a darkened room with a cool aromatherapy compress on the forehead.

Consider homeopathy. This is probably a safer alternative than herbs, especially for very young children. Children rarely need the most potent remedies, so for self treatment stick to 6c potencies and give one tablet every half hour for up to four hours during headache attacks until the pain begins to ease. Try *Valeriana officianalis* or *Passiflora* to induce sleep and relieve anxiety; *Chamomilla* to calm frayed nerves, *Kali bromatum* for fearfulness and nervousness; *Carbo veg* or *Silica* for digestive disturbances; *Pulsatilla* for weepiness and changeability; or *Calc phos* for headaches caused by emerging teeth.

Using Relaxation

Children are as prone to stress as any of us. Studies into relaxation techniques have had variable results, but the overall trend is positive. In one American study, children who were diagnosed as suffering from tension headaches used a combination of relaxation and biofeedback to help the children's headaches. In this study more than half of the children experienced at least a 50 per cent improvement in the frequency and severity of their headaches. Other studies have shown similarly good results.

Harness the Power of Imagination

Visualisation and meditation can be useful in children who are still comfortable with using their imagination. Simple relaxation skills can be taught by parents at home.

Sit quietly with your child and ask him or her to imagine they are in a warm shower and that everywhere the water strikes their bodies instantly feels more relaxed. Stay with this image for as long as it takes for your child to feel relaxed. A similarly helpful guided image is to suggest that your child picture stepping into a warm pool where the water gradually rises over his or her toes, feet, ankles and gradually upwards. Ask your child to imagine that as the water touches their body, their muscles gently relax and their pain floats away. This is a form of progressive muscle relaxation which children will find less boring than formal progressive relaxation (and it's a good guided imagery for adults too).

Inevitably some parents and children will feel awkward about taking time to relax. It is amazing how little patience we have for doing 'nothing'. Don't nag your child if they don't do the exercises on their own. Talking to your child about headache pain and the benefits of learning to relax is a better approach. Better yet, if you want to try and get your child to use relaxation techniques, practise with them. It will probably do you both good.

You can further help by structuring space and time in the day for your child to relax. Instead of forcing your child to relax (which of course defeats the purpose!), let him or her know that this is something important they should want to be doing for themselves — and make it clear that you want to help them succeed. Most children will go along with this because it gives them control over the situation.

Further Investigation

In one of the most thorough trials to date on children's headaches, food allergy and the frequency of migraine, conducted by the Department of Neurology at London's Great Ormond Street Hospital and published in the medical journal *The Lancet* in 1983, researchers discovered that ninety-three per cent of the children in the trial — children who suffered from severe, frequent migraine — recovered once the foods they were allergic to had been detected and eliminated from their diet. The most common allergens are the same as those listed in Chapter 5.

Sleep

A recent study in a professional journal dedicated to the study of pain, showed that children's headaches can be caused by a variety of some simple, obvious factors. Chief among these were fatigue and lack of sleep. Fatigue and sleep deprivation were also leading causes of both tension and migraine headaches in the Finnish research discussed earlier.

To help your child sleep well, you can use gentle remedies such as sprinkling lavender oil on their pillows. Another good way to help your child unwind before bed is to have a warm bath with soothing essential oils in it. Make sure that the hour or so before bed is always quiet time and be as firm and regular about bed times as you can be. Although most children will balk at one time or another about bedtime, the more it becomes a routine, the less trouble they will have dropping off.

Charts

1. HEADACHES AT A GLANCE		
TYPE OF HEADACHE	*WHAT KIND OF PAIN?*	*MAIN SYMPTOMS*
Tension	Steady, dull aching. Builds up gradually. Like a band around the head.	Spreads from the back of the neck, to the whole head. Head feels heavy. Does not usually throb.
Migraine	Generally one-sided, centred above or behind one eye. Pulsating, throbbing — often in time with the pulse. Drilling. Can last 2 to 72 hours.	Moderate to intense pain. Tingling in hands and face, nausea and vomiting. Classic migraine is preceded by an aura with visual disturbances. Balance and mental function are affected.
Cluster	Stabbing, one-sided. Similar to migraine. Individual attack lasts 15 minutes to 3 hours.	Comes in cycles over a period of days. Pain is behind one eye with reddening and weepiness in that eye. Facial flushing, drooping eyelids, sweating, nasal congestion.

1. HEADACHES AT A GLANCE continued

BROUGHT ON/MADE WORSE BY	*BEST TREATMENTS*
Straining the neck and shoulder muscles. High blood pressure, stress of any kind, poor posture, food intolerance and allergy, long car journeys, computer work.	Acupuncture, aromatherapy, chiropractic, dietary and environmental changes, homeopathy, hypnotherapy, osteopathy.
Activity, light, loud noises, stress, food intolerance or allergy, hormonal changes, physical activity, car journeys, strong smells and musculoskeletal problems.	Acupuncture, aromatherapy, chiropractic, dietary and environmental changes, herbal medicine, homeopathy, hypnotherapy, osteopathy.
Seasonal changes, food intolerance and allergy, hormonal imbalance, alcohol, restless sleep and smoking.	Acupuncture, chiropractic, diet and environmental changes, herbal medicine, homeopathy, osteopathy.

1. HEADACHES AT A GLANCE continued

TYPE OF HEADACHE	WHAT KIND OF PAIN?	MAIN SYMPTOMS
Sinus	Comes on gradually. Pain is dull, aching, throbbing or gnawing.	Pressure in the forehead or behind the eyes and nose. Sinus area feels tender. Occasionally fever.
Trauma	Stabbing, sharp or dull and aching pain.	Usually at the site of trauma. Can be hard to distinguish from a tension or migraine headache. Moodiness, dizziness, nausea, insomnia, fatigue, reduced concentration.
Sensitivity/ Allergy	Generalised head pain which can be dull, aching or throbbing. Continuous or in waves.	Pain can be anywhere on the head or all over.

1. HEADACHES AT A GLANCE continued

BROUGHT ON/MADE WORSE BY	*BEST TREATMENTS*
Inflammation or infection in the sinuses. Food intolerance and chemical sensitivity, pollen, dust and smoke. Psychological stress. Occasionally musculoskeletal problems and changes in atmospheric pressure will contribute.	Acupuncture, aromatherapy, chiropractic, dietary and environmental changes, herbal medicine, osteopathy.
Brought on by a blow to the head. But can be referred pain from another bodily injury, especially in the spinal and neck area.	Acupuncture, chiropractic, homeopathy, osteopathy.
Food intolerance or allergy, chemical sensitivity, stress, hormonal imbalance.	Acupuncture, dietary and environmental changes, herbal medicine, homeopathy.

1. HEADACHES AT A GLANCE continued

TYPE OF HEADACHE	WHAT KIND OF PAIN?	MAIN SYMPTOMS
Rebound	Comes in steady jolts. Throbbing pain can be similar to migraine.	Usually the whole head. Can begin at back of neck and spread to entire head or to just one side.
Eyestrain	Like a tension headache. Mild steady pain. Can be felt as a pressure on the top or around the head.	Commonly located in the forehead and face. Occasionally at the back of the head or neck.
Dental	Dull steady pain, usually felt as pressure on the top of the head. There may be a clicking sound in the jaw.	Usually on both sides of the head, like a tight band around the head. Tenderness around the jaw and mouth.
Exertion	Sharp, throbbing pain which comes on suddenly.	Can be generalised or localised anywhere in the head.

1. HEADACHES AT A GLANCE continued

BROUGHT ON/MADE WORSE BY	*BEST TREATMENTS*
Overuse of pain medications, prescription drugs and stimulants such as caffeine, MSG and artificial sweeteners. Psychological stress, food intolerance or allergy, chemical sensitivity.	Acupuncture, dietary and environmental changes, herbal medicine, homeopathy, hypnosis.
Overuse of eyes, made worse by metabolic imbalances, emotional/psychological stress, hormonal imbalance. Occasionally digestive disturbances or musculo-skeletal problems.	Acupuncture, aromatherapy, dietary and environmental changes, homeopathy, osteopathy.
Faulty bite, tooth decay, gum infections, grinding the teeth at night. Pain sensations can be made worse in those who are run down or under pressure.	Acupuncture, chiropractic, corrective dentistry, homeopathy, hypnotherapy, osteopathy.
In sensitive individuals any activity such as aerobics, sex, coughing, a bowel movement or running can be a trigger. Metabolic imbalance and stress aggravate the problem.	Acupuncture, aromatherapy dietary and environmental changes, herbal medicine, homeopathy.

2. EVERYDAY REMEDIES

Over the years, many different folk remedies have evolved to give quick relief to headache pain. Some are more effective than others and while these will not address the root cause of your headache, they may help to ease the pain and get you back on track quickly. You may have to experiment to find the remedy which suits you best.

Many of the ingredients are those which you have to hand at home.

Brush Your Hair
Brushing your hair each day isn't just a vanity. It can help to improve the circulation in your scalp and reduce the occurrence of headache. Use a natural bristle brush or one with rounded tips and brush your hair in a downward motion. You can also give yourself a mini-massage by brushing in small circles, beginning at your temples and working your way down your scalp. Make sure you cover all of your scalp in this way for the greatest benefit.

Make a Compress
Cool and warm compresses on the head can be very restful and revitalising. All you need is a washcloth and a few ingredients commonly found in the kitchen. Soak your washcloth in one of the three following mixtures. Combined with a twenty-minute rest, this should help lift your headache.

Ginger Compress
Cut and peel one whole root of fresh ginger. Boil it in 3 cups of water until it turns cloudy. Soak your washcloth in the warm mixture and then apply it to the back of your neck. This works to expand the contracted muscles and relieve dull, steady pain.

2. EVERYDAY REMEDIES continued

Vinegar Compress
Soak your washcloth in vinegar and place it in the refrigerator until it is sufficiently chilled. Apply to your forehead, neck and temples. You can also inhale vinegar for quick relief. To do this, boil equal parts of vinegar and water; pour the mixture into a bowl or basin; place a towel over the bowl and your head and inhale the beneficial steam.

Herbal Compress
Almost any aromatic herb tea can be good for this, but ideally you should boil 3 cups of water and pour it over 1 tablespoon of lavender and 1 tablespoon of camomile. Steep for 20 minutes. Soak your washcloth in the mixture, wring it out and apply on the back of the neck and/or forehead. This mixture is equally effective warm or cool.

Treat Your Feet
Draw congestion away from your head with a warming foot bath. Put 1 tablespoon of powdered mustard or ginger in a basin big enough for both of your feet. Fill the basin with water as hot as you can bear; sit in a comfortable chair and slowly immerse your feet in the water. You can drape a towel over the basin to keep the heat in. Placing a cool washcloth on your forehead or neck will also help.

Alternatively, try an icy foot bath. Fill a basin with icy water and soak your feet in it. After a few minutes, your feet will start to feel warm and your headache may drain away.

Hot and Cold
Alternating hot and cold showers will help improve your circulation and avert the vascular type headaches caused by the

2. EVERYDAY REMEDIES continued

dilation and then constriction of the blood vessels. You should aim to do this each day, or better yet, twice a day for two or three months to help improve your circulation.

If you are away from home and can't jump into a shower, try alternating hot and cold water on your wrists. If you do this as soon as you feel a headache coming on, it may avert a full-blown headache.

Make a Tonic

There are two effective tonics commonly used for headache sufferers. The first is made from small pieces of ginger root, coriander seeds and diced garlic. Put these in a pan, bring to the boil and keep boiling until half the liquid is gone. What is left is a concentrated mixture which you can sip periodically throughout the day. Sweeten with honey if you prefer.

For headaches caused by digestive imbalances, an apple cider vinegar tonic can be helpful. Apple cider vinegar (be sure not to use any other kind) is pH neutral and has a long history of use in folk medicine. You can make a simple tonic of a glass of water with 2 teaspoons of apple cider vinegar added to it. Have this each day with 2 teaspoons of honey to follow if you prefer.

Go Nuts

Try eating a handful of unpeeled almonds. They contain the natural 'aspirin' salicin, a remedy which is used in areas of North Africa and Asia where almond trees are common.

Relief in a Bag

Some people find relief from breathing into a paper bag for fifteen or twenty minutes. The carbon dioxide you inhale when breathing your 'old' air can help avert vascular headaches. Try to lie down for twenty minutes afterwards, especially if you feel dizzy.

Useful Addresses

General

Institute for Complementary Medicine *and*
The British Register of Complementary Practitioners (BRCP)
P.O. Box 194, London SE16 1QZ. Tel. 0171 237 5165.

British Complementary Medicine Association (BCMA)
249 Fosse Road South, Braunston, Leicester LE3 1AE.
Tel. 0116 282 5511.

Acupressure

Shiatsu Society
Suite D, Barber House, Storey's Bar Road, Fengate,
Peterborough, Cambridge PE1 5YS. Tel. 01733 758341.

Acupuncture

British Acupuncture Council
Park House, 206-8 Latimer Road, London W10 6RE.
Tel. 0181 964 0222.

British Medical Acupuncture Society
Newton House, Newton Lane, Lr Whitley, Warrington,
Cheshire WA4 4JA. Tel. 01925 730727.

Alexander Technique

Society of Teachers of the Alexander Technique (STAT)
20 London House, 266 Fulham Road, London SW10 0EL.
Tel. 0171 351 0828.

Aromatherapy

International Federation of Aromatherapists
2–4 Chiswick High Road, Stanford House, London WY 1TH.
Tel. 0181 742 2605.

International Society of Professional Aromatherapists (ISPA)
ISPA House, 82 Ashby Road, Hinckley, Leicestershire LE10 1SN.
Tel. 01455 637987.

Chiropractic

British Chiropractic Association
Blagrave House, 17 Blagrave Street, Reading, Berkshire
RG1 1QB. Tel. 0118 950 5950.

Environmental Medicine

British Society for Mercury Free Dentistry
225 Old Brompton Road, London SW5 0EA. (Send SAE).

**British Society of Allergy, Environmental and Nutritional
Medicine**
P.O. Box 7, Knighton LD7 1WT. (Send SAE.)

Herbalism

National Institute of Medical Herbalists
56 Longbrook Street, Exeter EX4 6AH. Tel. 01392 426022.

**International Register of Consultant Herbalists and
Homeopaths**
32 King Edward Road, Swansea SA1 4LL. Tel. 01792 655886.

Homeopathy

British Homeopathic Association
27a Devonshire Street, London W1N 1RJ. Tel. 0171 935 2163.

Society of Homeopaths
2 Artizan Road, Northampton NN1 4HU. Tel. 01604 621400.

Hypnotherapy

British Hypnotherapy Association
67 Upper Berkeley Street, London W1H 7DH.
Tel. 0171 723 4443.

Nutrition

Society for Promotion of Nutritional Therapy
P.O. Box 47, Heathfield, East Sussex TN21 8ZX.
Tel. 01435 867007.

Institute for Optimum Nutrition
13 Blades Court, Deodar Road, London SW15 2NU.
Tel. 0181 877 9993.

Soil Association
86 Colston Street, Bristol BS1 5BB. Tel. 0117 929 0661.
(organic food and farming information)

Osteopathy

General Osteopathic Council
Osteopathy House, 176 Tower Bridge Road, London SE1 3LU.
Tel. 0171 357 6655.

Osteopathic Information Service
As above.

Stress Management

Centre for Stress Management
156 Westcombe Hill, Blackheath, London SE3 7DH.
Tel. 0181 293 4114.

Yoga

British Wheel of Yoga (BWY)
Central Office, 1 Hamilton Place, Boston Road, Sleaford,
Lincolnshire NG34 7ES. Tel. 01529 306851.

Further Reading

Brotoff, Dr Jonathan and Gamlin, Linda, *The Complete Guide to Food Allergy and Intolerance*, London: Bloomsbury 1998.

Colbin, Annemarie, *Food and Healing*, New York: Ballantine 1996.

Cummings, Stephen and Ullman, Dana, *Everybody's Guide to Homeopathic Medicines*, London: Gollancz 1986.

Galland, Leo, *The Four Pillars of Health*, New York: Random House 1997.

Galland, Leo, *Superimmunity for Kids*, London: Bloomsbury 1989.

Hoffman, David, *The New Holistic Herbal*, Shaftesbury: Element 1994.

Lockie, Dr Andrew, *The Family Guide to Homeopathy*, London: Hamish Hamilton 1989.

Lockley, Dr John, *Headaches: The Complete Guide to Relieving Headaches and Migraine*, London: Bloomsbury 1994.

Mansfield, Dr John, *The Migraine Revolution: the New Drug-Free Solution*, London: Thorsons 1986.

Milne, Robert and More, Blake, *The Definitive Guide to Headaches*, California: Future Medicine Publishing 1997.

Murray, Michael T. and Pizzorno, Joseph, *An Encyclopaedia of Natural Therapies*, London: Optima 1990.

Petty, Dr Richard, *Migraine and Headache: Treating the Whole Person*, London: Unwin 1987.

Shealy, C. Norman, *The Illustrated Encyclopaedia of Healing Remedies*, Shaftesbury: Element 1998.

Steinman, David and Samuel Epstein, *The Safe Shoppers Bible*, New York: Macmillan 1995.

Worwood, Valerie Ann, *The Fragrant Pharmacy*, London: Bantam 1997.

Index